ADVANCE PRAISE FOR
STRUGGLE AND SOLIDARITY:
SEVEN STORIES OF HOW AMERICANS FOUGHT FOR THEIR MENTAL HEALTH THROUGH FEDERAL LEGISLATION

"The authors of *Struggle and Solidarity* narrate stories that mark some of the most important milestones in the history of American mental health, and the prowess of the editorial team—Dr. Michael T. Compton and Dr. Marc W. Manseau—shines through in comprehensive yet succinct chronological chapters that make for an easy read. It is hard to set down the book once you start reading it—it is logical and flows easily, and you find yourself coming away from each chapter, unique in its own content, having learned a lot by putting pieces of history together. A remarkable amount of work has gone into decoding and studying the various laws and eloquently elucidating the events and circumstances that led to their enactment. The book shows how history, advocacy, and politics collectively wove the tapestry of the societal structures in which Americans lived, learned, and worked, and created and then sought to address racial and ethnic divides.

After setting the stage in the first chapter by informing readers how federal laws affect basic social determinants and thus directly mental health, the authors take us chapter by chapter through the stories behind seven major federal laws. Interspersed are pictures of the tireless advocates who dedicated a significant chunk of their lives to enacting these laws, and illustrations that depict change spanning decades. The book beautifully wraps up with a concluding chapter summarizing the lessons one can learn from history, with an unmissable commentary on systemic racism.

The concept is brilliant, the organization immaculate, the presentation uniform, and the execution seamless. Let us use the knowledge contained in this book to inform policies and drive the change that the American public is in desperate need of today. The book is a must-have for just about any bookshelf in any American household."

Sanya Virani, M.D., M.P.H., *Forensic Psychiatry Fellow, Alpert Medical School at Brown University, and American Psychiatric Association Resident-Fellow Member Trustee*

"The stories in this volume are presented in fascinating and engaging vignettes about ordinary people and their struggle for dignity and a better life. Social needs such as freedom from poverty, food insecurity, climate change, racism, and exploitation are elaborated to draw the reader to an inevitable conclusion. Mental health suffers because of these preventable social determinants. Policy-level change is imperative for impacts on large populations. This is a must-read historical review for anyone interested in advocating for the rights of populations and improving mental health."

Vivian B. Pender, M.D., DLFAPA, President, American Psychiatric Association, and Clinical Professor of Psychiatry, Weill Cornell Medical College

"This volume provides a fascinating historical journey into federal legislation of the United States and the impact these legal decisions have had on social determinants of mental health. The authors help us to step out of the medical model of treating illness and into a better understanding of how social factors must be addressed to gain and maintain mental health.

The authors begin by introducing the reader to Jack Geiger, M.D., and his lifelong dedication to treating the whole person, in their community, rather than just focusing on illness. This first chapter sets the stage for the remaining ones, which eloquently retell the history of significant legislation that had impacts on each of several identified social determinants of mental health. The chapters cover farming and access to food, labor and employment, income security, clean air, civil rights, education, and housing. The authors of each chapter describe the impacts of the legislation on these social and environmental systems and the resulting effect the laws had on public and individual mental health.

In each chapter, the balance between fiscal, political, and social needs is played out through the advocacy of great leaders and affected communities. This book tells the story of social rights, or lack thereof, and it is a must-read for mental health providers, policy makers, and advocates."

Stephanie Le Melle, M.D., M.S., Director of Public Psychiatry Education and Associate Professor of Clinical Psychiatry, Columbia University Medical Center, New York State Psychiatric Institute

"Drs. Compton and Manseau and the many chapter authors have done the field of psychiatry and the world of mental health an extraordinary favor by removing our blinders and locating us in the world we inherited and can help to recreate. They take the concept of *health in all policies*, no doubt obscure to many, if not most, psychiatrists, and firmly locate it in the historic actions of passionate advocates for change. Beginning with a eulogy for Dr. Jack Geiger, a leading activist physician of the past 60 years, they then lead us through the dramatic stories of seven legislative victories outside of health care, from the Agricultural Adjustment Act of 1933 to the creation of the Department of Housing and Urban Development in 1965, that changed American lives, including their mental health, for the better. Their argument is simple: When faced with societal challenges to their health, mental health, and well-being, regular Americans have found ways, through legislation and policy, although not always perfect, to move forward. It is tempting to ask if there is a need for psychiatry and psychiatrists to join these efforts. Compton and Manseau make a convincing argument that our profession's voice matters. They point to the emerging concept of mental health impact assessments and the need for psychiatric input in policy development. In the challenging world we live in, we have a choice to be silent or to follow the example of those before us who struggled to make it better. The stories in *Struggle and Solidarity* represent an excellent launching point for psychiatry's renewed engagement with our society and its future."

Kenneth S. Thompson, M.D., Medical Director, Pennsylvania Psychiatric Leadership Council

STRUGGLE AND SOLIDARITY

Seven Stories of How Americans Fought for Their Mental Health Through Federal Legislation

STRUGGLE AND SOLIDARITY

Seven Stories of How Americans Fought for Their Mental Health Through Federal Legislation

Edited by

Michael T. Compton, M.D., M.P.H.

Marc W. Manseau, M.D., M.P.H.

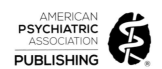

AMERICAN
PSYCHIATRIC
ASSOCIATION
PUBLISHING

If you wish to buy 50 or more copies of the same title, please go to www.appi.org/specialdiscounts for more information.

Copyright © 2023 American Psychiatric Association Publishing

ALL RIGHTS RESERVED

First Edition

Manufactured in the United States of America on acid-free paper
26   25   24   23   22   5   4   3   2   1
ISBN 978-1-61537-238-6 (paperback), 978-1-61537-405-2 (ebook)

American Psychiatric Association Publishing
800 Maine Avenue SW, Suite 900
Washington, DC 20024-2812
www.appi.org

Library of Congress Cataloging-in-Publication Data
A CIP record is available from the Library of Congress.

British Library Cataloguing in Publication Data
A CIP record is available from the British Library.

Contents

Contributors

Taiwo P. Alonge, M.D., M.P.H.
Adult Psychiatry Resident, Department of Psychiatry, Yale University School of Medicine, New Haven, Connecticut

Caroline L. Bersak, Esq.
Director of Legal Services, Legal Wellness Institute, The Family Center, Brooklyn, New York

Flávio Casoy, M.D.
Private practice, Brooklyn, New York

Michael T. Compton, M.D., M.P.H.
Professor of Psychiatry, Columbia University Vagelos College of Physicians and Surgeons; Research Psychiatrist, New York State Psychiatric Institute, New York, New York

Brie A. Garner, M.P.H.
Senior Project Manager, Housing for Health, NYC Health+Hospitals, New York, New York

Elizabeth Haase, M.D.
Associate Professor of Psychiatry, Department of Psychiatry and Behavioral Sciences, University of Nevada School of Medicine at Reno, Reno, Nevada; Medical Director of Psychiatry, Carson Tahoe Regional Medical Center, Carson City, Nevada

Jacob M. Izenberg, M.D.
Assistant Clinical Professor, Department of Psychiatry and Behavioral Sciences, University of California, San Francisco, California

Benson S. Ku, M.D.
Assistant Professor, Department of Psychiatry and Behavioral Sciences, Emory University School of Medicine, Atlanta, Georgia

Marc W. Manseau, M.D., M.P.H.
Clinical Assistant Professor of Psychiatry, Department of Psychiatry, New York University Grossman School of Medicine, New York, New York

Daniel Neghassi, M.D.
Assistant Clinical Professor of Medicine, Center for Family and Community Medicine, Columbia University Vagelos College of Physicians and Surgeons, New York, New York

Rebecca A. Powers, M.D., M.P.H.
Adjunct Clinical Associate Professor, Stanford University School of Medicine, White Oak Medical Office, Campbell, California
Email address for complimentary book ordering information:

Julie C. Suarez, M.A.
Associate Dean for Land-Grant Affairs, College of Agriculture and Life Sciences, Cornell University, Ithaca, New York

Andrew T. Turk, M.D., A.M.
Associate Professor, Department of Pathology and Cell Biology, Columbia University Vagelos College of Physicians and Surgeons, New York, New York

Matthew Wolfe, B.A., M.A., M.Phil.
Doctoral candidate, Department of Sociology, New York University, New York, New York

Disclosures

The following contributors have indicated that they have no financial interests or other affiliations that represent or could appear to represent a competing interest with their contributions to this book:

Taiwo P. Alonge, M.D., M.P.H.; Caroline L. Bersaq, Esq.; Flávio Casoy, M.D.; Michael T. Compton, M.D., M.P.H.; Brie A. Garner, M.P.H.; Elizabeth Haase, M.D.; Jacob M. Izenberg, M.D.; Benson S. Ku, M.D.; Marc W. Manseau, M.D., M.P.H.; Daniel Neghassi, M.D.; Julie G. Suarez, M.A.; Andrew T. Turk, M.D., A.M.

Foreword

Although steady advances in treatments for mental illnesses and substance use disorders are undoubtedly helping countless Americans, we must strive to promote well-being, mental health, and resilience in addition to offering treatment. To do this, with a goal to reach all Americans, *policy* must be a key part of the strategy. And policy with the farthest reach is that enacted by the U.S. Congress.

Recent decades have witnessed a recognition in the field of public health of *health in all policies*, meaning that health is created (or damaged) by many factors beyond the health care system and even beyond the traditional public health infrastructure. Health is shaped largely by the social determinants of health. As such, health-promoting policymaking across sectors—as diverse as education, energy, environment, farming and food, housing, labor, and transportation—in addition to the public health and health care sectors, can improve the health of all Americans. Relatedly, *mental health in all policies* means that there are hidden mental health impacts, either positive or negative, in all policies because they affect the social determinants of mental health. But how can we collectively influence the social determinants of mental health? One of the most powerful ways to shape these social and environmental factors in order to improve the mental health of millions of Americans is to ensure that policymaking takes such impacts into consideration.

The authors of this book tell the stories of seven major federal laws that had (mostly positive) mental health impacts "hidden" in plain sight, and which have largely gone unconsidered. These case studies make vivid the idea that policies, whether within an institution, an organization, local government, state government, or, in this case, federal legislation, can have far-reaching and long-lasting effects on mental health. Improving mental health and reducing the risk of mental illnesses and substance use disorders require smart, thoughtful, and rigorously analyzed and implemented policies. Furthermore, getting such policies passed legislatively and implemented well requires enormous efforts—often over decades—of everyday Americans, fighting for the conditions in work and life that would allow them, their families, and future generations a better, happier, and healthier future. The authors tell these stories of *struggle and solidarity* through key pieces of twentieth-century federal legislation.

Throughout my career in psychiatry and public health, I have witnessed the power of policy in promoting health and reducing risk of physical illnesses and behavioral health disorders. When I was a senior policy fellow and lobbyist for the Barton Child Law and Policy Clinic at the Emory University School of Law, we worked hard—in part through legislative advocacy—to improve measures that protect children from abuse and neglect. In my administrative duties as Medical Director of the Fulton County Department of Behavioral Health and Developmental Disabilities and as Director of the Fulton County Department of Health Services, I helped leverage state, local, and agency policy to improve the integration of public health, behavioral health, and primary care services as a means of improving access to care for all, but especially for those who had struggled most with access. In my elected roles—as president of the Georgia Psychiatric Physicians Association, Trustee of the American Psychiatric Association, Trustee of the American Medical Association (AMA), and, eventually, as President of the AMA—legislative advocacy was a necessary and crucial tool for advancing the health of populations. When I was Chair of the AMA Council on Legislation, the health impacts of federal legislation took priority.

We can make America healthier, with improved well-being, fewer psychosocial stressors, reduced structural determinants of health inequities, and longer and more meaningful lives. One key way to accomplish this is to fight for and pass laws and other policies that have beneficial, not detrimental, mental health impacts for all Americans. By demonstrating how Americans have worked together to improve mental health in the past, this book helps show us the way forward to a brighter, more equitable, and healthier tomorrow.

Patrice Harris, M.D., M.A.
Co-Founder and Chief Executive Officer, eMed
Former President of the American Medical Association

1 | Fixing the "Endlessly Revolving Door"

How Laws Impact Social Determinants and Thus Mental Health

Marc W. Manseau, M.D., M.P.H.
Michael T. Compton, M.D., M.P.H.

Pioneer in Social Medicine

In 1967, Dr. H. Jack Geiger—a primary care physician, Tufts University medical school professor, and civil rights activist—obtained funds from President Lyndon B. Johnson's Office of Economic Opportunity and combined them with private grants to start the nation's first community health center in Mound Bayou, Mississippi, a largely Black, rural, sharecropping community. He envisioned that clinic as not only providing medical care for the poor but also helping them with the social and economic problems that made them sick in the first place. In a 1970 short film, *Out in the Rural*, about the founding of the community health center, Dr. Geiger remarked that he was uninterested in "the idea that you stand around in whatever circumstances laying hands on people in the traditional medical way, waiting until they're sick, curing them and then sending them back unchanged into an environment that overwhelmingly determines that they're going to get sick" (Rogers 1970). The clinic used its federal and private funds to set up a library, a farming cooperative, and educational services, as well as other social supports.

Dr. Geiger also "prescribed" food to the malnourished children who came to the clinic for medical care, using clinic funds to pay for it. The governor of Mississippi complained to the federal government about this practice, and officials were sent from Washington, D.C., to admonish Dr. Geiger about a misuse of federal funds. Jack Geiger's response, now legendary within public health and social justice circles, was "Yeah, well, the last time I looked in my medical textbooks, they said the specific therapy for malnutrition was food." The federal officials returned to Washington without further interference in the project.

Shortly thereafter, Dr. Geiger used the same model to open the nation's first urban community health center in the Columbia Point neighborhood of Boston. This community health center model eventually expanded into a nationwide network of 1,300 clinics, providing health care and social services to more than 28 million low-income individuals at more than 9,000 sites, representing one of the most successful and lasting legacies of President Johnson's War on Poverty (Grady 2020).

Jack Geiger's interest in how social factors influence health did not come from a sudden epiphany in the Mississippi Delta, but rather from a lifelong commitment to social justice, formed during early life experiences. He was born Herman J. Geiger on November 11, 1925, in Manhattan, New York, and his childhood home on the Upper West Side hosted numerous Jewish relatives after they fled Europe to escape the emerging Nazis. He exceled as a student in New York City's public school system, skipping multiple grades and graduating high school at 14 years old. Too young to start college, he worked as a copyboy for *The New York Times* by day and attended jazz clubs in Harlem by night. He eventually became bored and frustrated and ran away from home, landing at the Harlem home of Canada Lee, a Black actor on Broadway whom he had met after a show he had attended. With Geiger's parents' permission, Mr. Lee took Jack in and let him stay in his living room for a year, where Jack met thinkers and artists, including Langston Hughes, Richard Wright, Adam Clayton Powell Jr., and Orson Welles. During this time, Jack listened as Lee's Black guests recounted various horrors of racism, including the mistreatment of Black troops at Southern military bases (Glass 1997; Grady 2020).

With a loan from Lee, Jack enrolled in college at the University of Wisconsin in Madison at 15 years old, where he quickly became involved in civil rights activities and started a chapter of the Congress of Racial Equality (CORE). He worked as a reporter for a local newspaper in the evenings.

Before he could graduate, however, he volunteered for the war effort by enlisting in the merchant marines, which he chose because it was the only branch of the military that was not racially segregated at the time. After World War II ended, in his early twenties, he decided that he wanted to combine his interests in health and social justice by pursuing a career in medicine, and he enrolled at the University of Chicago to complete his premedical studies. He continued his civil rights work with the CORE chapter there, protesting discriminatory treatment of Black patients at the hospital, as well as the rejection of qualified Black applicants by the medical school, which culminated in a large faculty-and-student protest strike. His activism led the American Medical Association to write a letter to medical schools across the United States warning them of his "extracurricular activities." As a result, he was unable to gain admission to any medical school; he was essentially blackballed from the medical field for his social justice work (Grady 2020).

Geiger returned to journalism for the next 5 years, working as a science and medicine editor for the International News Service. Through this job, he had the opportunity to meet with deans of medical schools, and he was eventually able to convince Case Western Reserve's medical school in Cleveland, Ohio, to admit him. Always academically precocious before this, he began medical school relatively late at 29 years old. During his fourth year, he traveled to South Africa to help set up and work at a health center in an impoverished Zulu reserve, Pholela. The health center not only provided medical care but also employed local people, built latrines, planted vegetable gardens, and ran malnutrition programs for children, among other nonmedical community development activities. It was there that he developed the ideas that would later become the community health center model in the United States (Brown and Benjamin 2021; Grady 2020).

Dr. Geiger decided that he wanted to go into international medicine, and he trained in internal medicine at Boston City Hospital and obtained a master's degree in epidemiology at the Harvard School of Public Health. However, his continued civil rights work showed him that there were poor people who needed his medical expertise and public health perspective right in the United States. He helped found the Medical Committee for Human Rights in the 1960s, an organization that provided medical care to frontline civil rights activists, including those who marched with the Reverend Dr. Martin Luther King Jr. from Selma to Montgomery in 1965. He also participated in the Freedom Summer in 1964, during which activists traveled on buses to the South in order to support the fight for civil and voting rights. It was during these experiences that Dr. Geiger realized that he did not need to travel to Africa to find deeply impoverished people in need of medical care and social services (Brown and Benjamin 2021; Grady 2020).

Dr. Geiger did not limit his lifelong advocacy work to civil rights in the United States. In 1961, he cofounded and led Physicians for Social Responsibility (PSR), which argued that the government was downplaying the health consequences of nuclear war and that physicians had an ethical responsibility to help prevent such earth-shattering devastation from happening. He presented at numerous professional meetings about the damage that a megaton nuclear bomb would do to the meeting's host city (called *the bombing run*). He also coauthored one of the first journal articles about the medical consequences of nuclear war, which appeared in *The New England Journal of Medicine* in 1962, just months before the Cuban Missile Crisis (Sidel et al. 1962). International Physicians for the Prevention of Nuclear War, of which PSR is a member, won the Nobel Peace Prize for this work in 1985.

In 1986, Dr. Geiger founded (and then led) Physicians for Human Rights (PHR), an organization that lent medical expertise to investigations of human rights violations across the globe and provided medical and social services to victims of human rights abuses. In 1997, the International Campaign to Ban Landmines, of which PHR is a member, won the Nobel Peace Prize for its work to ban landmines (Grady 2020; Physicians for Human Rights 2020).

Role of Policy in Shaping the Social Determinants of Mental Health

Although Dr. Geiger was a pioneer and master in leveraging the expertise and power of the medical field to turn knowledge about the social determinants of health into action, public health experts and social scientists have long recognized the central importance of social factors in determining health outcomes, a trend that has been accelerating. More recently, the importance of the social determinants of mental health has also gained traction (Compton and Shim 2015; Shim and Compton 2018). The social determinants are simply defined as "the conditions in which people are born, grow, live, work, and age," which can have powerful effects on the physical and mental health of both individuals and populations (World Health Organization 2018). Mental health effects of adverse social determinants include impairing people's ability to achieve optimal mental health and well-being, increasing the risk of mental illnesses and substance use disorders within populations, worsening outcomes for individuals with mental illnesses, and creating mental health inequities across groups. There are myriad well-established risk factors for mental illnesses, including, but not limited to, certain behaviors (e.g., drug and alcohol use), adverse experiences (e.g., childhood trauma), environmental exposures (e.g., in utero inflammation, parental mental illness, lead exposure), chronic stress responses, and genetics. The social determinants can be thought of as the "causes of causes" (Rose 1992) or the "fundamental causes of disease" (Link and Phelan 1995) and are themselves created out of an underlying unfair and unjust distribution of opportunity within society (Compton and Shim, 2015; Shim and Compton 2020). Examples of specific social determinants of mental health include adverse early life experiences, racism and other forms of discrimination, poor education and educational inequality, job insecurity and underemployment, poverty and income inequality, food insecurity, housing instability and poor housing quality, exposure to environmental toxins, and neighborhood deprivation.

As Figure 1–1 depicts, the social determinants of mental health stem from an unfair and unjust distribution of opportunity, and they lead to reduced behavioral options (and thus behavioral risk factors) as well as psychological and physiological stress, which in turn cause poor mental health outcomes as well as inequities in such outcomes. The social determinants of mental health are underpinned by two types of larger societal factors: public policies and social norms. Public policies are the official laws, regulations, and other policy decisions that govern how a society functions and distributes resources. Social norms are "the unwritten rules for how members of a society interact with one another," which can powerfully influence how opportunity and adversity are distributed (Shim and Compton 2018, p. 845). Public policies and social norms are themselves influenced by broad historical trends (e.g., a history of slavery and racial segregation in the United States), as well as overarching values (e.g., American values such as individualism, material comfort, and a belief in free market capitalism). Public policies and social norms also influence each other in a bidirectional manner, with laws shaping social norms over time and social norms determining the types of policies that a society will consider, prioritize, and ultimately enact.

Although recognition and scientific proof of the importance of social determinants have been growing steadily, public health and health care professionals have often struggled with how to intervene to improve them. Many have advocated for addressing the social determinants within health care settings, and programs to screen for them and then intervene through *social prescribing*—like what Jack Geiger did at community health centers and/or referring individuals with social needs to services that can support them—have shown promise (O'Gurek and Henke 2018; Roland et al. 2020). The instinct to attempt to intervene directly within health care is understandable for health care professionals and systems; however, confining attempts to improve the social determinants to health care settings has obvious limitations: people seeking treatment in health care settings are, by definition, more likely to already have the illnesses that one would have

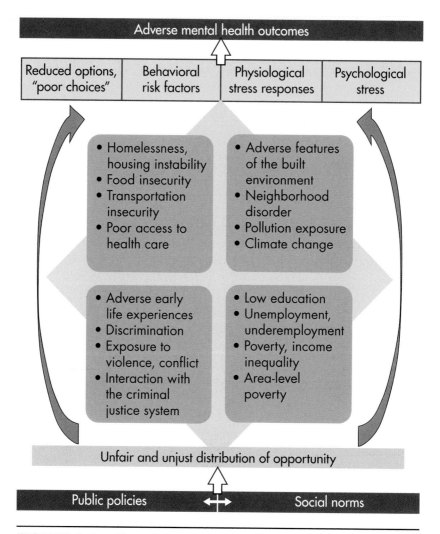

FIGURE 1-1. Conceptual model of the social determinants of mental health.

Source. Reprinted from Shim RS, Compton MT: "The Social Determinants of Mental Health: Psychiatrists' Roles in Addressing Discrimination and Food Insecurity." *Focus (American Psychiatric Association)* 18(1):25–30, 2020. Copyright © 2020 American Psychiatric Association Publishing. Used with permission.

wanted to prevent, not everyone has ready access to regular health and mental health care, and the health and mental health systems are designed primarily to provide treatment and not to improve underlying social conditions in society. Furthermore, the United States spends more on health care per capita (although less per capita on social services) than other wealthy nations but has worse health outcomes (Papanicolas et al. 2019), a problem that can never be fixed within the health care system itself.

Beyond the systems that directly provide physical health and mental health care, community interventions have been shown to effectively address social determinants and improve health and mental health outcomes. Examples include early childhood education programs such as Head Start (Barnett 1998; Schweinhart et al. 2005) and Nurse-Family Partnership (i.e., nurse home visiting) programs (Olds 2006). However, although such programs can effectively mitigate the negative impacts of adverse social determinants of mental health, they often cannot alter the underlying social determinants themselves. Only changes to policies and social norms hold the power to broadly improve the social determinants of mental health within society. Health and mental health professionals receive considerable public trust and have power within society and therefore have the potential to influence both policies and social norms (Shim and Compton 2018).

Seven Stories That Demonstrate Mental Health in All Policies

Calls to advocate for policy change and to influence social norms to improve the social determinants of mental health beg the question, How best can health and mental health professionals answer these calls? General entreaties to speak out, educate the public, and meet with elected officials, although well-intentioned, can at times seem vague to the point of being frustrating rather than motivating. High-impact advocacy work can be so complex and varied that a lengthy and detailed manual instructing health professionals on how to do it would likely be necessary. This book takes a different approach; it aims not to direct mental health professionals on what to do, but rather to tell the real-life stories of individuals and groups of people in the United States over the past century who succeeded in changing policies and vastly improving the social determinants of mental health. In essence, this book does not aim to *tell* readers how to advocate for policy change in the future but instead to *show* readers how others have successfully advocated in the past. Specifically, this book tells the stories of seven pieces of federal legislation enacted during the twentieth century that have had massive effects on the social determinants of mental health and have thereby improved mental health on a population level within the United States. Each chapter brings the argument to life that policies can have a substantial impact on the mental health of an entire nation by telling the stories of these laws in direct, vivid, and personal ways, drawing the real human experiences out of them. Although each chapter also devotes some space to reviewing the literature connecting the relevant social determinants of mental health to specific mental health outcomes, the goal is not to compile comprehensive reviews of the literature or bombard the reader with study designs and data points. Rather, the goal of each chapter is to give the reader a sense of what life in the United States was like without the given law, why the law was needed, the hard (and often dangerous) work of individuals and/or groups of Americans who got it passed, what the law actually did, and how it affected (and continues to affect) mental health. Each chapter ends with a look to the future because no law is perfect and the pursuit of better population mental health is never fully complete.

Readers might notice a few patterns in the book that may seem odd at first glance. For instance, all seven highlighted laws were enacted in either the 1930s or the 1960s. Further, all seven were signed into law by two Democratic presidents, President Franklin D. Roosevelt (as part of the New Deal) and President Lyndon B. Johnson (as part of the Great Society). Although important pieces of federal legislation were certainly left out (examples of which are described below), we opted for a sampling of the key twentieth century laws that had the largest and most enduring impacts on the social determinants of mental health. It just so happens that most of this fundamental legislation occurred during discrete periods of the twentieth century, and there are reasons for this. Progress in American federal policy has not advanced in an organized, linear fashion. Rather, it has tended to occur rapidly after tipping points, with decades of policy stagnation (e.g., the Gilded Age of the late nineteenth century) or even regression in between (e.g., the period after Civil War Reconstruction leading to Jim Crow). The conditions leading to these tipping points are described in many of the chapters.

Rapid progress tends to occur during and/or after periods of great crisis and desperation (e.g., the Great Depression), when radical change seems to be the only viable option, as well as during periods of revolutionary cultural transformation, when a critical mass of interests aligns and serves to organize large swaths of society toward change (e.g., the civil rights movement and anti–Vietnam War protests of the 1960s). This pattern may be due to the fact that large shifts in policy are difficult by design in the American democratic system and therefore tend to occur only when the same party controls the executive and legislative branches. In addition, as described in many chapters, powerful entities (e.g., corporate lobbyists, industry leaders) within the U.S. political-economic system often use their resources to block any progress that might threaten their interests, so the large amounts of energy and coordination necessary to counter these forces are possible for only short periods of time under special political and cultural conditions (Morone 1998).

Given that we focus on only seven laws, at least a few pieces of twentieth-century federal legislation might seem to be glaring omissions. For instance, the law creating the Medicare and Medicaid programs, signed by President Johnson in 1965, is left out here, despite obvious implications for the social determinants of mental health and immeasurably large benefits for the health and mental health of generations of Americans. The reason for this editorial decision is that a central goal of this book is to demonstrate how laws that seemingly have little to do with health or health care can have large impacts on health and mental health through their effects on non-health-care-related social determinants.

We also do not include, for example, a chapter on the Americans with Disabilities Act (ADA), signed into law by Republican President George H.W. Bush in 1990. This chapter could have told the story of how for 28 straight days in 1977, up to 200 people with disabilities continuously occupied the federal building in San Francisco—where offices of the then U.S. Department of Health, Education, and Welfare were located—in order to protest the watering down of regulations that the U.S. Department of Justice's Office of Civil Rights had written to protect individuals with disabilities from discrimination (thus demonstrating the need for separate legislation to achieve this aim) (Cone 2021). This chapter also could have told the story of the 1990 Capitol Crawl, when activists with physical disabilities dispensed with their various assistive devices and crawled up all 100 steps of the U.S. Capitol Building while Congress was in session, in support of the passage of the ADA (Eaton 1990). This chapter could have described how the ADA reduced discrimination against and promoted inclusion of (a key social determinant of mental health) individuals with disabilities across the entire country, vastly improving countless lives and bolstering mental health. The implications of the ADA for individuals living with mental illnesses—especially serious mental illnesses—are obvious.

In order to include laws that affect all Americans and therefore affect social determinants of mental health for the entire population, we focus on federal laws, even though countless state and local laws also have a great impact on mental health. Policies at the state and local levels—for which advocacy efforts may be successful—have significant and enduring impacts on the daily lives and therefore the mental health of Americans.

We also chose not to focus on state, federal, or Supreme Court decisions; presidential executive orders; or constitutional amendments. Judicial decisions (especially decisions by the U.S. Supreme Court) can have substantial effects on the social determinants of mental health. Consider the 1954 *Brown v. Board of Education of Topeka* decision, which banned racial segregation in U.S. schools, and the 2015 *Obergefell v. Hodges* decision, which gave equal access to the institution of marriage to all Americans regardless of their sexual orientation or the gender of their spouse. These and other court decisions have created or changed policies that have improved the mental health and well-being of large groups of Americans, acting through the social determinants.

Executive orders have also at times conferred substantial and long-lasting mental health benefits on the U.S. population. An outstanding example is President Abraham Lincoln's Emancipation Proclamation in 1862, which declared that all enslaved people in the states of the Confederacy "shall be then, thenceforward, and forever free," ending one of the most violent and traumatizing institutions the modern world has ever known. The Thirteenth Amendment to the U.S. Constitution then codified this ban on slavery (and "involuntary servitude") into the highest law of the nation, and the Fourteenth Amendment guaranteed due process and equal protection under the law to "all persons born or naturalized" in the United States, importantly including formerly enslaved persons. The importance of this executive order followed by these two constitutional amendments to the health and mental health of the American people cannot be overemphasized, and in fact, the Fourteenth Amendment provided the legal foundation for many subsequent pieces of progressive legislation, including the Civil Rights Act of 1964 (see Chapter 6, "Still on the Road to Freedom"). In 1919, about 50 years after the adoption of the Fourteenth Amendment, women's suffragists won their long fight for voting rights with the adoption of the Nineteenth Amendment to the U.S. Constitution. Providing full access to this pillar of American democracy to more than half the population who had been previously deprived of the right to vote improved multiple social determinants of mental health (e.g., social inclusion and discrimination, political power) for generations of American women, set the stage for further advances in women's rights, and likely made the enactment of many or even all of the laws described in subsequent chapters politically possible.

Although no chapter in this book focuses primarily on activities of the judicial or executive branches of the federal government, all chapters provide reference to key court decisions and presidential activities when relevant to telling the stories of the federal laws of interest. Having had to draw lines somewhere in order to craft a coherent book, we chose to organize the chapters around the activities of the most participatory branch of the federal government, the legislative branch. The legislative process is easier for everyday Americans to influence (i.e., it is more *participatory*) because legislators are regularly and directly elected (and reelected or not) by the people they represent and laws are passed much more frequently than, for instance, constitutional amendments (which are much more difficult to enact than laws and therefore much rarer). Although some local judges are elected, federal judges, including Supreme Court justices, are appointed, and the public has little opportunity to influence their decisions. Organizing the book around legislation therefore allowed the authors not only to demonstrate the importance of policies to the social determinants of mental health but also to tell compelling stories of everyday Americans actively working to improve their life conditions (and thus mental health).

Seven Laws That Improved Mental Health in a Big Way

Each of the following seven chapters tells the story of a major federal legislative act, and the chapters progress in chronological order by the year and month each law was enacted. These stories are generally structured to describe 1) the conditions in society that led to a groundswell of public interest, reaching the level of a societal crisis that had to be addressed; 2) one or more of the central figures—among the many—involved in the advocacy leading to the passage of the act; 3) a summary of the law itself; 4) evolution of the law over time, through reauthorizations and amendments; 5) the ways in which the federal law affected mental health in America (by affecting specific social determinants of mental health); and 6) shortcomings of the law and promise for future improvements. Specific figures are highlighted—whether they be academics turned policy experts such as Rexford Tugwell, seasoned politicians such as Edmund Muskie, or common Americans committed to taking up a cause for change (such as Harry Bridges, Esther Brown, and Oliver Brown)—to show that anyone can be involved in major policy change and thus can improve societal problems (and, even if inadvertently, the nation's mental health).

In Chapter 2, "Saving Farmers and Striving for Food Security," Compton and Suarez tell the story of the Agricultural Adjustment Act of 1933 (the first Farm Bill), one of the first policy moves undertaken by President Franklin D. Roosevelt to ease the agony of the Great Depression. The authors describe how a brilliant academic from New York, Rexford G. Tugwell, joined Roosevelt's Brains Trust and helped craft this revolutionary piece of legislation. They also argue that the first Farm Bill and its many subsequent revisions have reduced food insecurity in the United States and thereby improved the mental health of the American people. In Chapter 3, "From Worker Exploitation to Union Solidarity," Casoy and Manseau illustrate how the National Labor Relations Act of 1935 gave workers the right to organize and form labor unions, allowing them to push for better compensation and improved job conditions in a meaningful way for the first time in U.S. history. They tell the story of how generations of labor activists fought and even died for this basic right and how the ability to organize workplaces has improved mental health by addressing several social determinants of mental health, including those related to inequality, income, employment conditions, and power differentials within U.S. society. In Chapter 4, "Stay Against Financial Catastrophe," Bersak and Wolfe describe how Frances Perkins became the first female member of a presidential cabinet as President Roosevelt's Secretary of Labor and how she used that position to help design and push for passage of the Social Security Act of 1935. The authors argue that this act became the foundation for all subsequent federal welfare legislation and in this way had a massive impact on economic social determinants of mental health, including poverty or low income, and income inequality.

In Chapter 5, "Clearing the Air for Mental Health," Ku and Haase tell the story of how a lifelong environmental warrior, Senator Edmund Muskie of Maine, successfully fought for one of the most important and impactful pieces of legislation to protect the environment and therefore our health and mental health, the Clean Air Act of 1963. The authors describe how the act and its subsequent revisions have reduced air pollution by almost unfathomable amounts and review data linking air pollution to poor mental health outcomes, showing how this act has vastly improved America's mental health. They also discuss the potentially catastrophic mental health implications of climate change and show how the Clean Air Act may provide a foundation for viable solutions going forward. The discussion in Chapter 6, "Still on the Road to Freedom," centers on the Civil Rights Act of 1964, and Neghassi and Alonge vividly describe how Black activists such as Ella Baker fought with passion, sweat, and blood against Jim Crow and for a society that would treat all people with dignity and equality. They demonstrate how social determinants such as racism and racial inequity harm mental health and how the Civil Rights Act moved toward successfully mitigating this harm within American society. They also argue that although the United States has made significant progress since the 1960s, racism remains entrenched within American society, and they discuss possible future solutions. In Chapter 7, "The Times They Are A-Changin'," Powers describes the Elementary and Secondary Education Act of 1965, emerging out of major culture changes in the 1960s, when outright educational inequality was finally no longer to be tolerated. With the stage set by Esther Brown in Merriam, Kansas, and Oliver Brown in Topeka, Kansas, in the 1940s and 1950s, it was not until 1965 that Congress acted to ensure that all children should have access to high-quality education. Finally, in Chapter 8, "Remodeling and Breaking New Ground," Izenberg et al. tell the story of the Housing and Urban Development Act of 1965 and place this act within the context of overall American housing policy. Although the authors discuss how this act meaningfully improved the social determinants of housing stability, quality, and equity in the United States and thereby improved mental health outcomes, they are critical in general of U.S. policy around housing. Indeed, this history is characterized more by failure than by successes, but they end on a hopeful note when describing practical solutions for the decades-long contemporary U.S. housing crisis. All seven of the laws, although promoting mental health, had serious weaknesses that would have to be dealt with in iterations over the decades following their passage—and in the years to come following publication of this book.

Yet Another Call to Action

Dr. H. Jack Geiger died on December 28, 2020, at age 95 (Grady 2020). Early in his career, in 1969, he wrote the following, which now seems both clairvoyant and just as true as it was then:

> Right now we health professionals are standing in the middle of an endlessly revolving door…doing some good on a short-term basis…. [But] we cannot go on providing health services without regard to the system in which the roots of poverty, sickness, and many other social ills are embedded. We have to be willing to identify the real problems and confront them…we have to create new social institutions appropriate to the problem; and, finally, we need a sense of passionate commitment to bring about the changes that are so urgently needed. (Brown and Benjamin 2021, pp. 792–793; Geiger 1969)

The door still endlessly revolves, and it sometimes seems that we have barely begun to address the roots of poverty and sickness in the United States. But Dr. Geiger's life set a hopeful and inspiring example. He maintained the "sense of passionate commitment to bring about the changes that are so urgently needed" that he described in 1969 for the rest of his life. He deserves his place in the proud legacy of all the passionate activists, fervent social justice fighters, and visionary policy thinkers whose stories this book tells.

We need more people like Jack Geiger in the mental health and medical fields and in society (Figure 1–2). We need more people who are brave and clear-eyed enough to endure personal and professional sacrifice to advocate for social justice; that is the only way that the growing calls to address the social determinants will move from research and writing (as important as they are) to the action and change we so desperately need. As Geiger did, we must recognize that fundamental transformation, rather than incremental change and the tweaking of current systems, will be necessary if we are to make the United States a healthy and safe place where all people can thrive. And we must be willing to fight for this transformation.

We hope that this book demonstrates in a vivid and compelling way just how vital policy, specifically federal legislation, has been to the mental health of all people in the United States. We also hope that this book will

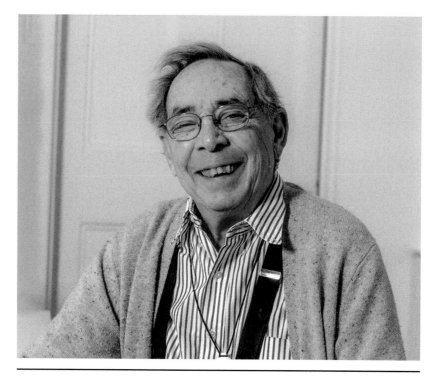

FIGURE 1–2.   **Dr. Jack Geiger at his home in Brooklyn, New York.**
Source. Copyright © 2016, Erin Patrice O'Brien Photography. Used with permission.

inspire people to get involved in pushing for social and policy progress, just like the individuals highlighted in these chapters did, and that it will show that fundamental change can occur within the American democratic system. At the time of this book's writing, the United States was struggling with multiple overlapping crises: a global pandemic with enormous morbidity and mortality tolls, economic stress for many amid unprecedented levels of inequality, threats to our democracy, and the specter of climate change. Although only hindsight will tell us for certain, the United States may be at another tipping point, when history shows us that there is so much promise of progress if we organize and advocate for it effectively.

References

Barnett WS: Long-term cognitive and academic effects of early childhood education on children in poverty. Prev Med 27(2):204–207, 1998 9578996

Brown TM, Benjamin GC: Dr. H. Jack Geiger, a towering public health leader. Am J Public Health 111(5):792–794, 2021 33826383

Compton MT, Shim RS (eds): The Social Determinants of Mental Health. Washington, DC, American Psychiatric Publishing, 2015

Cone K: Short history of the 504 sit-in. Berkeley, CA, Disability Rights Education and Defense Fund, 2021. Available at: https://dredf.org/504-sit-in-20th-anniversary/short-history-of-the-504-sit-in. Accessed August 20, 2021.

Eaton WJ: Disabled persons rally, crawl up capitol steps: Congress: scores protest delays in passage of rights legislation. The logjam in the House is expected to break soon. Los Angeles Times, March 13, 1990. Available at: www.latimes.com/archives/la-xpm-1990-03-13-mn-211-story.html. Accessed February 1, 2022.

Geiger HJ: Endlessly revolving door. Am J Nurs 69(11):2436–2445, 1969 5195307

Glass I: Kindness of strangers, in This American Life. National Public Radio, September 12, 1997. Available at: www.thisamericanlife.org/75/kindness-of-strangers. Accessed August 17, 2021.

Grady D: H. Jack Geiger, doctor who fought social ills, dies at 95. New York Times, December 28, 2020. Available at: www.nytimes.com/2020/12/28/health/h-jack-geiger-dead.html#:~:text=28%2C%202020-,Dr.,He%20was%2095. Accessed February 1, 2022.

Link BG, Phelan J: Social conditions as fundamental causes of disease. J Health Soc Behav Spec No:80–94, 1995 7560851

Morone JA: The Democratic Wish: Popular Participation and the Limits of American Government, Revised Edition. New Haven, CT, Yale University Press, 1998

O'Gurek DT, Henke C: A practical approach to screening for social determinants of health. Fam Pract Manag 25(3):7–12, 2018 29989777

Olds DL: The nurse-family partnership: an evidence-based preventive intervention. Infant Ment Health J 27(1):5–25, 2006 28640426

Papanicolas I, Woskie LR, Orlander D, et al: The relationship between health spending and social spending in high-income countries: how does the US compare? Health Aff (Millwood) 38(9):1567–1575, 2019 31411912

Physicians for Human Rights: Dr. H. Jack Geiger, founding member and a past president of PHR: a visionary advocate for health and human rights. New York, Physicians for Human Rights, December 29, 2020. Available at: https://phr.org/our-work/resources/dr-h-jack-geiger-founding-member-and-a-past-president-of-phr. Accessed August 18, 2021.

Rogers JS (dir): Out in the Rural: A Health Center in Mississippi. 1970

Roland M, Everington S, Marshall M: Social prescribing—transforming the relationship between physicians and their patients. N Engl J Med 383(2):97–99, 2020 32640128

Rose G: The Strategy of Preventive Medicine. New York, Oxford University Press, 1992

Schweinhart LJ, Montie J, Xiang Z, et al: Lifetime Effects: The High/Scope Perry Preschool Study Through Age 40. (Monographs of the High/Scope Educational Research Foundation, No. 14). Ypsilanti, MI, High/Scope Educational Research Foundation, 2005

Shim RS, Compton MT: Addressing the social determinants of mental health: if not now, when? If not us, who? Psychiatr Serv 69(8):844–846, 2018 29852822

Shim RS, Compton MT: The social determinants of mental health: psychiatrists' roles in addressing discrimination and food insecurity. Focus (Am Psychiatr Publ) 18(1):25–30, 2020 32047394

Sidel VW, Geiger HJ, Lown B: The medical consequences of thermonuclear war II: The physician's role in the post-attack period. N Engl J Med 266:1137–1145, 1962 13912536

World Health Organization: Commission on Social Determinants of Health: closing the gap in a generation: health equity through action on the social determinants of health. Final report. 2018. Available at: www.who.int/social_determinants/final_report/csdh_finalreport_2008.pdf. Accessed August 19, 2021.

2 | Saving Farmers and Striving for Food Security

The Agricultural Adjustment Act of 1933

Michael T. Compton, M.D., M.P.H.
Julie C. Suarez, M.A.

Collapse of Crop Prices, Famished Farmers, and Tons of Dust

The situation facing farmers during the Great Depression was nothing short of dire, and it involved growing too much, not growing too little. This seeming paradox is caused by the fact that farmers' sustenance and the sustainability of any farm depend to a great extent on crop prices. And crop prices in the early 1900s were at the root of the crisis for farmers. The golden years of

The authors are grateful for reviews, advice, and substantive input provided by Paul Alward at Veritas Farms, New Paltz, New York; Amy Ehntholt at New York State Psychiatric Institute, New York, New York; and Leah Pope at Department of Psychiatry, Columbia University Vagelos College of Physicians and Surgeons, New York, New York.

good prices for commodity crops were 1909–1914, a period that, as we will see, became a point of reference in our act of interest, the first Farm Bill, the Agricultural Adjustment Act (AAA) of 1933. *Commodity crops*, a focus of this chapter, refer to relatively nonperishable, storable, and transportable crops that are traded, such as wheat and dried field corn, and require processing before consumption or use. Today, such crops are what most large farms produce, in massive fields with very long rows cultivated and harvested with large machinery. The end uses of commodity crops include livestock feed, ethanol, flour, and food additives. As such, we are not talking about fruits and vegetables that have become known in the farming world as *specialty crops*, which tend to be more perishable depending on whether they are grown for the fresh or processing market and which return higher prices to the farmer while requiring greater skill and attention to the cropping system.

When World War I (1914–1918) severely disrupted agriculture in Europe, the American commodity crop farmer was able to substantially increase production and export surpluses across the Atlantic. In fact, the government encouraged expansion of farm output. The American frontier seemed to become one large wheat field. Although prices plateaued and the golden years did not last long, they would serve as a reference point during years when prices took a nosedive and emergency measures were needed to save farmers.

Everyone knows that when supply of a good exceeds demand for it, its price falls. This phenomenon was central to the farmers' problem, but just as multiple factors had brought about the Gilded Age, many events and practices converged to take farmers to the brink of starvation. By the 1920s, European agriculture had recovered, American farmers were having more difficulty finding export markets for their products, and surpluses resulted in falling prices. The boll weevil (a beetle) hit Southern cotton fields between about 1915 and 1925, destroying millions of acres. The 1920s saw many manufacturing and production booms, aided in part by increased demand for consumer goods (think flapper dresses made of rayon rather than cotton). Falling crop prices brought about difficulty paying farm mortgages and, eventually, serious financial problems for farmers. To add to the growing economic concern, farmland had become *overfarmed* (overcropping, overgrazing, constant tillage of the soil contributing to high rates of erosion)—depleted, dry, and dusty.

As the Great Depression set in across the country, crop prices fell not incrementally, but drastically. Indeed, the Great Depression itself decreased demand markedly across the economy for everything, including commodity crops, and this was a major reason in and of itself for plummeting crop prices (Conkin 1987). Farmers literally could not sell crops for more than it cost to grow them. The situation was dire, unprecedented, and even deadly. By 1932, prices were at an all-time low (Figure 2–1). Huge surpluses of commodity crops such as wheat and corn accumulated, yet many people were struggling to access enough food for their own families. It was reported that in South Dakota, for example, grain elevators had corn priced at minus three cents a bushel—it would cost a farmer three cents to sell a bushel of corn. Entire fields of cotton remained unpicked because its selling price was not worth the cost of labor. Wheat was being burned in lieu of coal because it was cheaper and had little or no market value. Farm families were starving, and thousands of their farms were abandoned.

As farmers had settled the plains and other areas of the country and moved away from subsistence farming to more modern commodity crop farming, their farms had become so specialized that they could not feed their families (one cannot eat cotton or only wheat). Subsistence farming had been a very hard life as the country settled, but the specialization that had developed in 1900s agriculture had resulted in prices being more robust in the buildup and aftermath of World War I (driven by increased demand from European countries for American-produced farm goods, given the devastation occurring in Europe) (Hall 1973). However, improved farming practices ultimately left farmers in a significant poverty and food insecurity bind when prices dropped. The onslaught of the Great Depression had many underpinnings, but it was generally agreed that economic conditions would not be righted until farming was brought back from collapse.

Although some farmers were organizing and protesting, others were quietly surrendering to foreclosure. William Hirth (1932), president of the Missouri Farmers' Association in Columbia, Missouri, summarized the situation in *The Billings Times* on Thursday, December 22, 1932:

> Then what of our farmers of America who at this hour owe approximately fifteen billion dollars upon which they are paying from 6 to 8% interest, and which interest must be met under the threat of foreclosure or the menace of the sheriff's hammer? And yet no one has heard a whimper about repudiation from these farmers—with long suffering patience as the collapse of farm prices has bitten in deeper and deeper, they have merely pointed out to the powers that be that they cannot meet these gigantic obligations with a 50c farm dollar, and especially so when during recent years practically one third of their yearly income has been required for taxes. And on top of this, since the World War our farmers have suffered a loss in land values of twenty billion dollars, or a sum equal to more than the value of our great American railroad system, and thus as one visualizes these tragic facts one realizes that our so-called farm problem is indeed an overshadowing one—either farm prices must be jacked up to assure our farmers of a generous purchasing and debt paying dollar, or the final and complete collapse of Agriculture is as certain as the rising and setting of the sun.

Farmers faced low odds of surviving. And then came the dust. Tons upon tons of topsoil blew off barren fields, creating smothering clouds of dust for hundreds of miles. Although the driest region of the Great Plains

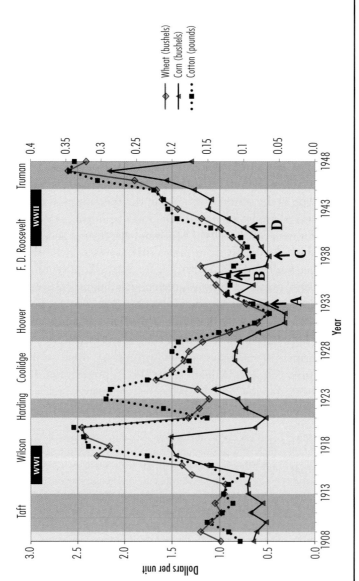

FIGURE 2-1.   Crash of commodity crop prices, culminating in 1932.

Wheat, corn, and raw cotton prices by unit from 1908 to 1948. The left *y* axis shows dollars per bushel for wheat and corn, and the right *y* axis shows dollars per pound of cotton. The bottom *x* axis gives the year, and the top *x* axis shows the president during the shaded time period. A=Agricultural Adjustment Act, 1933; B=Soil Conservation and Domestic Allotment Act, 1936; C=Agricultural Adjustment Act, 1938; D=Steagall Amendment, 1942.
Source.   Data from U.S. Bureau of the Census 1960.

(southeastern Colorado, southwest Kansas, and the panhandles of Oklahoma and Texas) became known as the *Dust Bowl*, nearly the entire country came to be affected. The invention of the first John Deere steel plow in the late 1800s, the availability of cheap federally subsidized prairie land, and a drive to rapidly settle the nation's expanding population set up conditions perfectly for the nation's most challenging environmental and agricultural natural disaster—the Dust Bowl. The rich, productive soil, formerly held together by woven mats of prairie grasses and sod during the inevitable cycles of drought and high winds, was no longer anchored but instead was tilled regularly every year by farmers industriously planting shallower-rooted commodity crops (Montgomery 2007, 2012).

In 1932, 14 dust storms blew formerly productive soil from the western half of the United States all the way to the U.S. Capitol Building in Washington, D.C.; there were 38 in the following year. Between 1930 and 1934, rainfall in Nebraska, to use just one state as an example, dropped by more than a quarter, resulting in corn crop yields plummeting by three-quarters. It was dry and dusty. Seeds blew out of the ground, porches and houses were constantly under a layer of dust, and there was not enough rain to offer even a few minutes of respite from the drifting dirt. The 1936 Soil Conservation and Domestic Allotment Act—and the AAA of 1938 (the second Farm Bill) and subsequent Farm Bills—would have to tackle this problem on the ground, but our attention here will focus on events leading to a momentous act in 1933, during President Franklin Delano Roosevelt's first 100 days.

Down-and-Out Farmers, a Rural Uprising, and Voluntary Domestic Allotment

Farms were failing, farm families were distraught, and the nation was spinning toward economic collapse. Such downward spiraling sometimes leads to an uprising, in this case not with swords or rifles, but with pitchforks and picket signs. The farm revolt of the early to mid-1930s has been described as *agrarian activism* and as a *rural insurgency*. It was a rising up of the farmers, who found themselves downtrodden and in the hardest of times: arid and dusty land, bottomed-out crop prices, and a country slumping deeper and deeper into economic and psychological depression. There are many stories to tell. Farmers' Holiday, for one, was when farmers went on strike and picketed in the roads leading to markets, spurred in part by the Communist-led United Farmers League. The Farmers' Holiday Association in Iowa, the Dakotas, and other Midwestern states had as its slogan "Stay at Home—Buy Nothing—Sell Nothing."

Newspaper headlines across the country read "Farmers and Police Clash at Iowa Highway Blockade" (1932), "Farmers Plan Protest Parade" (1932), and "Georgia Farmers Dump Milk" (1932). Farmers rallied other farmers to destroy their crops as a means of reducing supply and thereby attempting to raise prices, although it was unlikely to work given the economic condition of the country. There were "milk strikes" from the Midwest to upstate New York. The farmers had, in fact, been experiencing an agricultural depression throughout the otherwise "roaring" 1920s, but the situation had become dire after the stock market crash of 1929. The Agricultural Marketing Act of 1929 under the Hoover administration had attempted to stabilize prices by having the Federal Farm Board purchase, store, and sell surpluses, but it simply could not keep up with the excess production in the context of plummeting demand. Farm organizations (such as the American Farm Bureau Federation, the National Grange, and the Farmers' Union) unequivocally found the Hoover administration to be completely ineffective—useless, in fact. They needed a real "Farmers' President."

As the 1932 presidential campaign took shape, Roosevelt would hold promise as the Farmers' President. It comes through in his radio address from Albany, New York, from the parlor of the governor's executive mansion on July 30, 1932, while he discussed the Democratic Party platform (Roosevelt 1932):

> We advocate for the restoration of Agriculture, the nation's basic industry; better financing of farm mortgages through re-organized farm bank agencies, at low rates of interest, on an amortization plan, giving preference to credits for the redemption of farms and homes sold under foreclosure; extension and development of the farm-cooperative movement; and effective control of crop surpluses so that our farmers may have the full benefit of the domestic market.

In campaigning, he spoke of an unusual-sounding *voluntary domestic allotment* plan, which would ultimately be elaborated and enacted in the act that would be among the first and most influential programs of the New Deal. And it would be the first Farm Bill, which has since evolved drastically over the decades and forms the basis of the nation's agricultural policy to this day.

This economic approach to saving the farmers—domestic allotment or production control—had many early proponents, including economists William J. Spillman; John D. Black; Beardsley Ruml; and, perhaps most importantly, Milburn L. Wilson, a voting Republican who had been an agronomist (professor of agricultural economics) at Montana State Agricultural College and who had served at the U.S. Department of Agriculture (USDA) during the Coolidge administration (Badger 2008). Wilson, in fact, convened a conference of influential leaders, bankers, and economists on April

10, 1932, to develop the plan. Others privately opposed the concept of production control. For example, at one New York Ivy League institution, Cornell University, George Warren—another renowned farm economist also influential with Roosevelt (New York State College of Agriculture 1957)—believed that governmental restrictions on production for farmers were unworkable and that a more competitive marketplace was best in the long run, without a monetary system tied to the gold standard.

Although many men were involved, to ultimately make the AAA the law of the land, the next elected president would need a trusted adviser to work out the details. That man was neither an agrarian activist nor a rural insurgent; he was rather a young professor of economics at the other New York Ivy League institution, Columbia University in New York City. This man was Rexford G. Tugwell (Figure 2–2), who was a member of Roosevelt's *Brains Trust*, a group of about a dozen intellectuals (mostly university professors) assembled to advise the candidate on topics related to their various disciplines and help his bid for presidency. Tugwell had the needed smarts in the area of agricultural economics.

The Man Who Made It Happen: Professor Rexford G. Tugwell

Although many people were involved in the creation of the AAA—Henry Wallace, Henry Morgenthau, George Peek, and Hugh Johnson, among others—Rexford G. Tugwell found himself within the Brains Trust (which, as he describes in his book titled *The Brains Trust* [Tugwell 1968], was a term coined by *New York Times* correspondent James M. Kieran while he was covering the Roosevelt campaign) and thus had the ear of the candidate and, later, the president. Roosevelt was not regarded—by others or by himself—as an intellectual; his personality was his driving force. But he was always willing to listen to experts. During his approximately 4 years in the Roosevelt administration and throughout a long and circuitous career thereafter, Tugwell was viewed by many as a dedicated progressive and adherent of the visionary British political economist John Maynard Keynes. He and others in the Brains Trust were able to convincingly explain to Roosevelt and other administration officials how the Keynesian idea of *central planning* could make society stronger and more stable and that central planning was needed to pull the farmers out of the Depression. Although Roosevelt trusted his ideas, others would come to characterize Tugwell's approach as collectivist and extreme during a conservative backlash to the New Deal and Keynesian economic management, even casting accusations of anti-capitalism, if not communism (which was partly, although ludi-

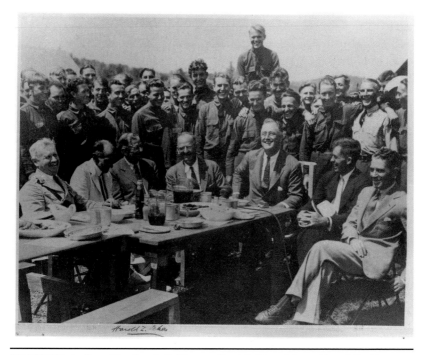

FIGURE 2–2.   Rexford G. Tugwell with President Franklin D. Roosevelt.

Photograph (August 12, 1933) of President Franklin D. Roosevelt with (*from left to right, seated*) General Paul Malone, Louis Howe, Harold Ickes, Robert Fechner, Henry Wallace, and Rexford Tugwell (*in the folding chair on the far right*). Standing are men of Civilian Conservation Corps (CCC) Company 350 at CCC Camp Big Meadows in the Shenandoah Valley of Virginia.
Source.   Franklin D. Roosevelt Presidential Library and Museum, Hyde Park, NY (public domain).

crously, linked by some to a 10-week trip to the Soviet Union made by Tugwell as part of a trade union delegation while he was at Columbia).

So what was Tugwell's story? Born July 10, 1891, in Sinclairville, New York, Rexford Guy Tugwell grew up immersed in an awareness of the importance of farming. Sinclairville is situated in Chautauqua County in western New York, about 60 miles south of Buffalo. Rexford's parents, Charles and Dessie, were strong supporters of progressive Democratic candidates (Namorato 1988). His father was an ambitious entrepreneur, engaging in the cattle business, orchard farming, canning, and banking. In his autobiography, *The Light of Other Days*, Tugwell (1962) described his father as "an enterpriser of the old-fashioned sort, always considering new ventures, turning his energies to whatever promised to yield a profit, and always, I may say, making money" (p. 76). As for his mother, she could not have been

more the opposite: no practical planner, Dessie was an intellectual and a ro-
mantic, and a doting mother. Tugwell described, "She was certain, for instance, that I was extremely talented in practically every kind of endeavor,
and she was just as insistent that I had been born truthful, honest, generous,
and kind" (Tugwell 1962, p. 78).

Having had a happy and privileged upbringing in rural New York,
Tugwell went on to study at the University of Pennsylvania's Wharton
School of Finance and Commerce. Positions followed at the University of
Washington, the American University of Paris, and Columbia University,
where from 1920 to 1932 he ascended the academic ranks from instructor
to full professor of economics. In 1932, Professor Tugwell was recruited,
along with two Columbia colleagues, Raymond Moley and Adolf Berle,
into Roosevelt's Brains Trust, during which time he became a central figure
in the crafting of the AAA. And indeed, Tugwell had the candidate's ear. As
Tugwell (1968) described in his *The Brains Trust*, after an evening of dinner
and deliberation at the executive mansion in Albany in April of 1932, Mrs.
Roosevelt called the discussions to a halt at midnight, after which Ray Moley
told Tugwell that Roosevelt had never listened to anyone for so long.

Although he would need to convince Roosevelt of the way forward on
the farming crisis, which would eventually become the AAA, in more general terms, Tugwell believed strongly in the role of central planning. The
theory was that capitalism causes instability—even of the magnitude that
led to the Great Depression—and that the solution for regaining stability
was through planning. In terms of agriculture, instability had grown from
an excess of competition across unaffiliated farmers, leading to overproduc-
tion of commodity crops. As growers continued increasing their production
and specialization, partly as a result of agricultural advances (such as tractors and other farm equipment) and in hopes of a higher financial return,
the increased supply did not create an increase in demand, as classical lais-
sez-faire theory about free markets predicted. Families need only so much
flour, cornmeal, rice, and milk (and furthermore could afford only so much
when unemployed during a depression). Tugwell saw central planning as
the solution to this poverty of relative abundance by creating a balance between production and consumption, with the linchpin being farmers' cooperation, ensured through promises of solvency from the government.

Agricultural Adjustment Act of 1933

Background

Roosevelt's first term began with remarkable efficiency. Many major,
groundbreaking pieces of legislation were enacted into law, representing an

enormous effort to pull the country out of economic depression. Roosevelt was inaugurated president on March 4, 1933, the last newly elected president to endure the excessively long waiting period between election and inauguration before the Twentieth Amendment (ratified on January 23, 1933) moved subsequent Inauguration Days to January 20. He soon called Congress into special session to introduce a record number of legislative proposals under what he dubbed the New Deal. Twelve days after inauguration, Roosevelt called on Congress to include relief for agriculture as part of the new series of emergency legislation (Kolb 1933). The first 100 days were probably the wildest and fastest 100 days Congress had ever—and possibly has ever—seen. The 26-page AAA was passed on

May 12, 1933. Some aspects of the new Farm Bill, as Roosevelt had called it, were counterintuitive, so the president explained the bill to the public himself. In his third fireside chat (his radio addresses from the White House) on the evening of Monday, July 24, 1933, the president spoke to Americans about the AAA of 1933 (Figure 2–3). There would be many letters to farmers and farming organizations in the months and years to come, in which this Farmers' President directly addressed leaders in New York State and U.S. farm communities.

A main component of the cure for farmers' economic woes was to not produce so much: voluntary domestic allotment. This innovative but controversial notion consisted of three elements: 1) acreage restriction, meaning reduced crop production and quotas; 2) taxes on the processing companies that processed agricultural commodities (e.g., turning wheat into flour and cotton into yarn); and 3) benefit payments, from the proceeds of those taxes, distributed to the farmers who cooperated with the production quotas. This was admittedly experimental. But desperate times called for unproven, even completely theoretical, policy measures. And the farmers would need help getting together—associating, collaborating, and making agreements—to bring total production down in order to see prices come up.

Before we get into the three titles of the act, a summary of the concepts is as follows: The basic intent of the AAA was to restore the purchasing power of American farmers to the pre–World War I levels of the golden age. The money to pay the farmers for cutting back production by at least 30% would be raised by a tax on companies that bought farm products and processed them into food and clothing. The AAA evened the balance of supply and demand for farm commodities so that prices would support a decent living for farmers. This concept was known as *parity*. But parity would not save the farmers; the act would also need to craft strategies for better financing of farms.

After the adjournment of the historical special session of the Congress five weeks ago I purposely refrained from addressing you for two very good reasons.

First, I think that we all wanted the opportunity of a little quiet thought to examine and assimilate in a mental picture the crowding events of the hundred days which had been devoted to the starting of the wheels of the New Deal.

Secondly, I wanted a few weeks in which to set up the new administrative organization and to see the first fruits of our careful planning.

I think it will interest you if I set forth the fundamentals of this planning for national recovery; and this I am very certain will make it abundantly clear to you that all of the proposals and all of the legislation since the Fourth day of March have not been just a collection of haphazard schemes but rather the orderly component parts of a connected and logical whole....

For many years the two great barriers to a normal prosperity have been low farm prices and the creeping paralysis of unemployment. These factors have cut the purchasing power of the country in half. I promised action. Congress did its part when it passed the farm and the industrial recovery acts. Today we are putting these two acts to work and they will work if people understand their plain objectives.

First, the Farm Act: It is based on the fact that the purchasing power of nearly half our population depends on adequate prices for farm products. We have been producing more of some crops than we consume or can sell in a depressed world market. The cure is not to produce so much. Without our help the farmers cannot get together and cut production, and the Farm Bill gives them a method of bringing their production down to a reasonable level and of obtaining reasonable prices for their crops. I have clearly stated that this method is in a sense experimental, but so far as we have gone we have reason to believe that it will produce good results.

FIGURE 2–3. **Excerpt from Franklin Delano Roosevelt's third fireside chat, given on Monday, July 24, 1933, at 9:30 P.M.**

Source. National Archives: Roosevelt's fireside chat on the recovery program, 1933. Available at: www.archives.gov/education/lessons/fdr-fireside. Accessed February 1, 2022.

The Act's Three Titles

The AAA, signed into law in the spring of 1933 in the depths of the Depression, begins with this straightforward but highly impactful introductory statement:

> An act to relieve the existing national economic emergency by increasing agricultural purchasing power, to raise revenue for extraordinary expenses incurred by reason of such emergency, to provide emergency relief with respect to agricultural indebtedness, to provide for the orderly liquidation of joint-stock land banks, and for other purposes.

The act stands on just three legs, three titles, each reliant on the others and briefly summarized below.

Title I: Agricultural Adjustment

Title I is perhaps the easiest of the three for a noneconomist to understand and may be the title that Rexford G. Tugwell had the greatest input into because it is a grand demonstration of central planning. The title begins with a "Declaration of Emergency." The acute economic emergency, as the act notes, was due in part to a *severe and increasing disparity* between the prices of agricultural and other commodities that had 1) destroyed the purchasing power of farmers for industrial products, 2) broken down the commodities markets, and 3) seriously disrupted agricultural assets (e.g., land loans) supporting the national credit structure. The act later defines the agricultural commodities of concern as the "basic crops" of wheat, cotton, field corn, hogs, rice, tobacco, and milk; as such, the act covered nearly all American farmers because no matter where in the country a farmer lived, chances were that farmer was growing in large part one of these named commodities.

After stating the emergency, the act then declared a basic policy approach ("Declaration of Policy"). The approach would be to establish and maintain a balance (known as *parity*) between commodity production and consumption—supply and demand—and in doing so, reestablish prices for farmers to a level that would give agricultural commodities a purchasing power with respect to the articles (such as tools and equipment) that farmers buy. But reestablishing prices to what level? Specifically, the act states that the "base period" would be the prewar, golden-years period of August 1909 to July 1914 (for tobacco, the base period would be August 1919 to July 1929). The concept of parity—embedded in all Farm Bills in some shape or another (albeit much modified in the 1960s and 1970s) until the Federal Agriculture Improvement and Reform Act of 1996, or Freedom to Farm Act—was groundbreaking in the farming community. Farmers were to be paid a percentage of what crop prices were in the boom years. Those boom years were modified over time, and eventually, the concept of parity became one of a percentage of payment based on what the world market prices were for the particular commodity.

Reestablishing equality of purchasing power would be done by a "gradual correction of the present inequalities therein at as rapid a rate as is deemed feasible in view of the current consumptive demand in domestic and foreign markets." In other words, the federal government would need to work urgently to address a crisis but would do so in a measured manner that the national and global economies could tolerate. And it would need to be done in such a way that consumers (Americans) could tolerate—the readjustment of farm production should not increase the percentage of citizens' retail expenditures for agricultural commodities (or else their hunger would be made worse). It would require a balancing act, and the act gave the soon-to-be-established Agricultural Adjustment Administration the leeway needed to do it.

In 1934–1935, the list of commodities being targeted was expanded to include others such as rye, flax, barley, grain sorghum, cattle, peanuts, sugar beets, sugar cane, and potatoes. Evidently, very few farmers refused to take the government payments; most could not afford to refuse, and most presumably understood the dire supply-demand dilemma they were in. The AAA affected about 99% of farmers of the time; it was less or not beneficial to smaller farms and subsistence farms, tenant farmers, and sharecroppers, a problem that we return to shortly.

Title II: Agricultural Credits

Title II, under the short title of the "Emergency Farm Mortgage Act of 1933," was an economically complex portion of the act that had a number of parts dealing with loans, interest rates, mortgages, and other aspects of the financing of farms. It made amendments to the Federal Farm Loan Act, for example, allowing federal land banks to issue farm loan bonds for the purpose of making new loans or for purchasing mortgages or exchanging bonds for mortgages. Mortgages were refinanced with terms more favorable to struggling farmers.

Title III: Financing—And Exercising Power Conferred by Section 8 of Article I of the Constitution: To Coin Money and to Regulate the Value Thereof

This title, also called the Thomas Amendment after Senator Elmer Thomas of Oklahoma, pertains to the president's authority, through his secretary of the treasury, to regulate the currency. Here, George Warren at Cornell was involved, despite his concerns about Title I. This financing facet of the act involves the Federal Reserve, and it involves silver and gold. The president could expand the currency through several mechanisms, such as printing greenbacks, reducing the value of the dollar relative to gold, and accepting silver as payment for European countries' World War I debts. Without the authorities provided by this title, the loan and mortgage provisions of Title II might not work, and without those provisions, the domestic allotment of Title I would likely not work. This approach, representing a massive break from past monetary management, would allow Roosevelt the financial flexibility to fund the New Deal.

Summary

On the AAA's passage in 1933, a planned national farmers' strike was called off, and meanwhile, Tugwell was appointed assistant secretary of agriculture (Roosevelt had asked him what post he would like) and then undersecretary of agriculture the following year. Together, he and the secretary, Henry Wallace, led the USDA in its implementation of the AAA's expansive authorizations (Badger 2008).

In general terms, the AAA accomplished a number of objectives. Perhaps most importantly, in a time of urgency, it gave broad emergency authority to the president, USDA, and Treasury and established the Agricultural Adjustment Administration. Through its various provisions and authorities, it restored the purchasing power of farmers to pre–World War I levels through voluntary domestic allotment, created means of refinancing mortgages with terms that were more favorable to struggling farmers, and provided the economic logistics and currency levers to make it all work. As we will see in the section "Importance of Economic Stability and Food Security for Mental Health," however, unbeknownst to the men creating the act, the AAA was also an important piece of mental health legislation—perhaps one of the most important pieces of mental health legislation—both during the Great Depression and in the decades since.

Rexford G. Tugwell Across the Years After the AAA

The man who made the AAA happen continued to have an impact in the Roosevelt administration and beyond. In 1935, while undersecretary of agriculture, Tugwell also took on the position of director of the Resettlement Administration (Conkin 1987). If the AAA is considered his first brainchild, programs within the Resettlement Administration were surely his second. In general, these programs aimed to relocate struggling urban and rural families to communities planned by the federal government. The Resettlement Administration, which set into stone Tugwell's thinking on the role of government in planning, cannot be seen as a political or planning success. It did, however, construct three *greenbelt* towns: Greenhills, Ohio, near Cincinnati; Greendale, Wisconsin, near Milwaukee; and the largest and best known, Greenbelt, Maryland, a Washington, D.C., suburb. Greenbelt, with its many art deco–style buildings, seen as a utopian experiment by some and a socialist advance by others, was an attempt by the federal government to build a self-sufficient, cooperative community for those needing housing while at the same time creating jobs and thus stimulating the national economy, similar to the Works Progress Administration and the Tennessee Valley Authority. The planning and construction of the greenbelt towns did not last long, however, because the one planned for New Jersey (Greenbrook) would bring the program to an end. The U.S. Court of Appeals for the District of Columbia found the program unconstitutional in *Franklin Township in Somerset County NJ v. Tugwell* (1936). It ruled that housing construction was a state power and that the Resettlement Administration was an illegal delegation of the Federal Emergency Relief Administration's power.

Through successes and failures, Tugwell believed that careful and well-informed governmental economic planning could reduce the instability of capitalism and improve living conditions for the citizenry. He advocated for more government control over business. He was opinioned in his ideologies around the role of government and was not prone to compromise—traits that made him controversial and a target for critics during his years in public life. In addition to his central role in crafting the AAA and leading the Agricultural Adjustment Administration within the USDA, Tugwell was instrumental in creating the Soil Conservation Service in 1933. This service aimed to help farmers restrict cultivation, restore poor-quality land, and introduce better agricultural practices for soil conservation in light of the devastation of the Dust Bowl of the 1930s. He also was integral in drafting the 1938 Federal Food, Drug, and Cosmetic Act, which authorized the FDA to oversee the safety of food, drugs, medical devices, and cosmetics.

After his years advising Roosevelt and serving in the USDA, Tugwell would continue on an interesting career trajectory, for example, as chancellor at the University of Puerto Rico (Namorato 1988). After leaving the Department of Agriculture in 1936, he served as the first director of the Planning Department of the New York City Planning Commission (appointed in 1938 by Mayor Fiorello LaGuardia). In 1942, he was appointed governor of Puerto Rico during World War II. He served as the last colonial governor appointed to that office, just as the citizens of Puerto Rico were given the power to elect their own public officials, and helped usher in Luis Muñoz Marín, the first elected governor.

Tugwell returned to teaching in 1946, becoming a professor of political science and the director of the Institute of Planning at the University of Chicago. He retired from the university (and from his ongoing work with the Caribbean Commission) in 1957 but remained active as a lecturer and writer. Among his 20 books were *A Chronicle of Jeopardy, 1945–55* (Tugwell 1955) on the decade since the atomic bomb attack on Hiroshima; *The Art of Politics, as Practiced by Three Great Americans: Franklin Delano Roosevelt, Luis Munoz Marin, and Fiorello H. LaGuardia* (Tugwell 1958); and *The Enlargement of the Presidency* (Tugwell 1960), in which he chronicles the accomplishments and shortcomings of the presidents and argued that the powers and functions of the office of the president had reached a limit too big for a single person and was in need of a "radical breakthrough" in which the office is reestablished as a plural executive. These were in addition to many books on Roosevelt; the New Deal; the Brains Trust; the policies of other presidents; and the role of economic, urban, and rural planning.

Tugwell died at 88 on July 21, 1979, at which time the Farm Bill was on its tenth iteration: the United States Food and Agriculture Act of 1977 (also known as the 1977 U.S. Farm Bill). Some 44 years after the passage of the original AAA, that Farm Bill continued policies to support farmers. It established, for example, a new two-tiered pricing system for peanuts (Jimmy Carter was president at the time): growers were given an acreage allotment on which a poundage quota was set. Growers could produce in excess of their quota within their acreage allotment but would receive the higher of the two price levels only for the quota amount. By this time, nutrition assistance programs were well established within the Farm Bill as the nation's key policy approach to addressing food insecurity (Imhoff 2012). In the 1977 bill, Title XIII was designated the Food Stamp Act of 1977, amending the Food Stamp Act of 1964 by simplifying eligibility requirements. Incrementally, since the devastating Great Depression, U.S. society could be more and more sure of the availability of its food. Tugwell's closeness to Roosevelt in 1933 clearly shaped the future of agricultural policy, rural land planning, and food security, and his relationship with the president in turn surely shaped what would become a fascinating and productive career and life story. In a final tribute to the relationship between the two men, Tugwell's papers—114 boxes of correspondence, diaries, speeches, writings, and memorabilia—reside at the Franklin D. Roosevelt Presidential Library in Hyde Park, New York, alongside those of the president.

Unconstitutionality and the Farm Bill Across the Decades

It could be argued that the voluntary element was the act's downfall because farmers could easily fallow land that was marginal for production and still receive the payment (thus, as George Warren at Cornell would have said, focusing just on acreage reductions and not yield quotas would not work). As efficiency and the land grant system of research and extension kept helping farmers to grow more and more food (i.e., more and more yield) per acre, the AAA's system as it was initially constructed was not sustainable in the end, regardless of the processing tax's ultimate demise on the grounds of unconstitutionality.

In 1936, the Supreme Court ruled the AAA unconstitutional, with Justice Owen Roberts writing for the majority that by regulating agriculture in such a way, the federal government was invading areas of jurisdiction reserved by the Constitution to the states; the AAA of 1933 thus violated the Tenth Amendment. It was deemed illegal to tax one group, the processors, such as those converting wheat into flour and cotton into yarn, in order to pay another group, the farmers. A new version of the AAA was enacted in 1938, addressing these problems by imposing marketing quotas and over-production penalties, rather than subsidies for farmers who limited production. The 1938 act was later upheld by the Supreme Court.

In the interim, in 1936, Congress enacted the Soil Conservation and Domestic Allotment Act, which helped maintain production controls by offering payment to farmers for trying new crops, such as soybeans. As evidenced by its name, this law enacted measures to combat the Dust Bowl, such as planting soil-conserving trees and native grasses. Crop insurance was included in the AAA of 1938, the second Farm Bill, which, as noted above, paid subsidies from general tax revenues instead of taxes on processors because of the Supreme Court's ruling. The 1938 act expanded support beyond the traditional commodity crops by introducing supports for butter, dates, figs, hops, pecans, prunes, and other farm products. Certain pulses (dry peas and dry beans), flaxseed and peanuts for oil, potatoes, sweet potatoes, and other products were included in the Steagall Amendment in 1942.

What began as emergency legislation would need to evolve to become meaningful policy during stable times while still being responsive when unforeseen downturns—economic, climatic, or otherwise—occurred. Usually on a 5-year cycle, the Farm Bill is revisited, and its various and expanding facets are redeliberated and renegotiated. In the deliberations, sometimes, regional battles are fought, pertaining to commodity production regions in the South (e.g., cotton), Midwest (e.g., corn), and Great Plains (e.g., sugar beets), and often, partisan concerns are at play (for example, in more recent decades, funding and eligibility for food and nutrition assistance programs for low-income households). Commodity interest groups and a host of food processing and manufacturing lobbyists are always at the table. The bill's scope has expanded, the number of various interested parties has grown, and compromise has become increasingly central to the success of reauthorization, especially during periods of a tightly divided Congress when bipartisanship is required.

By 1949, in Harry S. Truman's administration, the bill was amended to include rules for the donation of surplus food to friendly overseas countries and for the federal government's assistance to the states in establishing, operating, maintaining, and expanding school lunch programs. The Farm Bill was no longer just about farmers but was about the food security of the country's children. During Lyndon B. Johnson's administration, in 1964, the Food Stamp Act provided permanent legislative authority to the Food Stamp Program, which had been administratively implemented on a pilot basis in 1962. Food security of all Americans thus became a target of the

Farm Bill under Johnson and subsequent administrations. To some extent, the Farm Bill has always represented an uneasy tension between advocates for government assistance for food security and farm groups. This tension, or alliance between groups with different interests, seemed a healthy one because rural interests could not in and of themselves carry farm subsidy, crop insurance, and conservation programs and required urban legislators to also weigh in and support the food security aspects of the bill. In recent decades this partisan détente has often been part of the deliberation and re-authorization process. Although sometimes contentious, in most years, support for the Farm Bill has been one of the few instances in which a Republican and a Democrat from the same state would agree because of the context of the Farm Bill providing both food assistance to hungry people and farm subsidies.

In the Carter administration, in 1977, eligibility requirements for Food Stamps were simplified, and Title XIV was designated the National Agricultural Research, Extension, and Teaching Policy Act, which made the USDA the leading federal agency for agricultural research, extension, and teaching programs. Some iterations of the Farm Bill would have a greater or lesser focus on support to farmers with regard to peanuts, rice, milk, and even wool, as well as other commodity crops, depending on market vicissitudes and farmers' stability versus struggles.

In 1985, a dairy herd buyout program was put into place, taking entire milk-producing farms off-line, as yet another attempt to control production and pricing of milk. Although the USDA had been purchasing surplus dairy products through the Dairy Price Support Program, more drastic measures were needed. In 1984, a milk diversion program was established to pay farmers to reduce their milk marketings by 5%–30%, with about 38,000 dairy operations participating. However, success was minimal and short-lived, in part because nonparticipating dairy farmers expanded their production. Thus, a 1985 measure—milk termination and herd buyout—was designed to reduce the milk supply by removing dairy cows from production altogether. Some dairy farms converted to beef farms, and beef assumed an increasingly larger place on the American dinner plate. (It should be noted that one barrier to success was that after a period of time, some dairy farms that had sold their herds simply started anew, which was allowed under the dairy buyout. That is, after taking a break for a year and paying down debt, some farms restarted as a dairy again, which was not at all infeasible because they had all the equipment and it is not so hard to restart if all one needs are cows.) Like those related to wheat and corn in the 1930s, efforts to control milk production would evolve in Farm Bills over the years. Many would argue that the Farm Bill continues to be less successful in the dairy sector than for row crops, although the most recent 2018 Farm Bill's authorization of the Dairy Revenue Protection risk management tool, which allows farmers to insure against significant price declines, has shown promise and has significantly assisted many dairies facing financial disruption from the coronavirus SARS-CoV-2 disease (COVID-19) pandemic.

In addition to addressing the complex issues of supply, pricing, and demand, the Farm Bill's crop insurance provisions have evolved over the years, giving reassurance to farmers who might otherwise be sunk by multiple years of weather events and natural disasters. Crop insurance typically extends only to large farms; the small, local, organic vegetable farm would not be included in the program until the Farm Bills in 2014 and 2018 made significant improvements to specialty crop and whole-farm crop insurance, folding in smaller farm operations and including diversified fruit and vegetable farms that tend to be more heavily concentrated in the organic sector.

Built-In Inequities

During its brief existence, the original AAA, the first Farm Bill, accomplished its goal: the excess of commodity crops decreased, and prices rose. Farmers regained purchasing power. The act is considered by some to have been among the most successful programs of the New Deal. But the act was a product of white men, and consideration for the livelihoods of Black sharecroppers was missing from the development and, critically, the implementation of the AAA. As an unsurprising consequence, the law inordinately favored large landowners, and subsidies were distributed to landowners, not to sharecroppers, who were abundant in the South. Sharecroppers were poor farmers working the landowner's land and receiving a share of the crop at harvest time. When the landlords left their fields fallow because of production containment, sharecroppers were often left without work. Tractors and other emerging equipment were sometimes purchased by landowners with the subsidies, which exacerbated the job losses among sharecroppers because of the improved efficiency and mechanization strategies (White 2018). (This is but one example of a constant push-pull dynamic in agriculture related to simultaneously striving to improve working and living conditions and wages for farmworkers in an industry that is primarily seasonal while being able to compete with global open-trade conditions in agricultural commodities. Here, the advent of technology brought about labor efficiencies, which meant fewer people employed.) Under the AAA, although landowners had legal obligations to compensate sharecroppers and tenant farmers on their land, enforcement was lax or nonexistent. Tenant farmers rented the land, provided their own supplies, were given less supervision, and received half the crop. The number of tenant farmers in the South dropped drastically in the late 1930s, and the AAA may have played a role. By the time of the 1936 Soil Conservation and Domestic Allotment Act, landowners were required to share the payments they received from the government for reduced production with those who worked on their land.

Also implicated in built-in inequities are the harmful and egregious impacts of the Jim Crow laws that caused many Black-owned farms to fail in this time period, despite the development of innovative Black-owned agricultural cooperatives. Inadequate assistance from the USDA has been well documented and was particularly acute with the development of what is now known as the Farm Service Agency's local county, which had approval power over loans and loan guarantees and frequently discriminated against Black farmers (White 2018). This issue was central in *Pigford v. Glickman* (1999), a class action lawsuit against the USDA alleging racial discrimination against African American farmers in its allocation of farm loans and assistance between 1981 and 1996. Since the decision, nearly $1 billion has been paid or credited to thousands of farmers under the settlement's consent decree.

There is, nonetheless, a need to fully address and account for ongoing systemic inequities starting with the first Farm Bill for Black, Indigenous, and other disadvantaged farmers moving forward into future iterations of the Farm Bill. Issues of systemic discrimination and racism in agriculture are still being fought today. The inclusion in the 2021 American Rescue Plan of $5 billion in debt relief and financial assistance to Black, Indigenous, and People of Color (BIPOC) farmers was a significant recourse for generations of inequity, particularly because the USDA has indicated that less than 0.1% of COVID-19 farmer assistance funds had previously been allocated to BIPOC growers (Ducheneaux 2021; Vilsack 2021). However, nearly as soon as the USDA announced program implementation details, a lawsuit was filed in Wisconsin, and a stay was issued at the behest of white farmers who alleged discrimination. These issues add to the burden of mental health for BIPOC farmers; the typical stressors farmers face are exacerbated by the additional burdens of systemic racism.

Farm Bill Today and in the Future

The current version of the Farm Bill, the 530-page Agriculture Improvement Act of 2018 (compared with the 26-page AAA), became law on December 20, 2018, and provides for the reform and continuation of agricultural and other programs of the USDA through fiscal year 2023. Its 12 titles deal with a vast array of issues pertaining to farming and related activities:

1. Commodities, including commodity policy, marketing loans, sugar policy, dairy-related provisions, agricultural disaster assistance, and related policy
2. Conservation, including wetland conservation, the Conservation Reserve Program, the Environmental Quality Incentives Program, the Conservation Stewardship Program, and related programs and policy
3. Trade, including the Food for Peace program and agricultural trade laws
4. Nutrition, including the Supplemental Nutrition Assistance Program (SNAP), formerly the Food Stamp Program; commodity distribution programs; and related food security projects
5. Credit, including farm ownership loans and operating loans
6. Rural development, including programs to combat substance use disorders in rural America and connect rural Americans to high-speed internet and amendments to the Consolidated Farm and Rural Development Act
7. Research, extension, and related matters
8. Forestry
9. Energy, including bioenergy and biofuels
10. Horticulture, including organic certification policy
11. Crop insurance
12. Miscellaneous policies and programs

With regard to Title IV, on nutrition, within the Food and Nutrition Service of the USDA, more than a dozen federal nutrition assistance programs aim to increase food security and reduce hunger by providing children and low-income families with access to food, a healthful diet, and nutrition education in a way that supports American agriculture: SNAP; Special Supplemental Nutrition Program for Women, Infants, and Children (WIC); Farmers Market Nutrition Program; Senior Farmers' Market Nutrition Program; Child and Adult Care Food Program; National School Lunch Program; School Breakfast Program; Summer Food Service Program; Special Milk Program; Fresh Fruit and Vegetable Program; Food Distribution Program on Indian Reservations; Commodity Supplemental Food Program; and Emergency Food Assistance Program. These programs serve one in four Americans during the course of a year. SNAP alone reached 38 million people nationwide in 2019 (Foster et al. 2021), and recent efforts, often at the state and local levels, strive to steer more SNAP benefits toward fresh produce and healthier options. Despite the successes, 10.5% (13.8 million) of U.S. households were food insecure at some time during 2020 (U.S. Department of Agriculture 2021a).

Importance of Economic Stability and Food Security for Mental Health

So what does all of this have to do with mental health and mental illnesses in America? The AAA and subsequent Farm Bills have had major population-level impacts on at least two social determinants of mental health—the economic viability of farms and farmers (as well as that of entire rural communities where the local economy is centered on farming) and food security—and likely others. That is, although the Farm Bill started as a means of saving the farmers, it now extends to striving for food security for the nation.

The Farm Bill has sought to prevent economic hardship among farmers, especially those growing commodity crops and dairy products, for nearly a century. Between about 1928 and 1933, farmers saw rising taxes on their property; mortgage debt reached a perilous peak; and many farmers lost their farms because of the combination of decreased income, heavy taxes, and burdensome debt, as well as, in certain geographic regions, the disastrous consequences of the Dust Bowl. Foreclosures, defaults on taxes, and bankruptcies ensued. The 1933 AAA began a series of policy maneuvers, most notably boosting agricultural prices (putting money in the hands of farmers) by reducing surpluses, to prevent this overproduction-related facet of the Great Depression from ever happening again. Farm income in 1935 was more than 50% higher than farm income during 1932 (Rasmussen et al. 1976). In alleviating poverty and associated food insecurity, the Farm Bill also improved mental health for farmers and their families.

Although farmers may have been the primary focus of the original Farm Bill, given the decline in farming as an occupation, modern Farm Bills likely have a greater impact on nonfarmers. According to the USDA, after peaking at 6.8 million farms in 1935, the number of U.S. farms fell sharply until the early 1970s. More recently, the number of U.S. farms has continued to decline, but at a slower pace. As of 2019, there were 2.02 million U.S. farms, and the average farm size was 444 acres (U.S. Department of Agriculture 2021b). Corn and soybeans accounted for 43.1% of the total crop cash receipts in 2019, with vegetables accounting for only about 9.8%. Median total household income among all farm households is about $83,000, and most households earn some income from off-farm employment. About half of U.S. farms are very small, with annual farm sales under $10,000; the households operating these farms typically rely on off-farm sources for most of their household income (U.S. Department of Agriculture 2021b).

The AAA, in conjunction with other acts during Roosevelt's first term, was designed to pull the country out of the Great Depression by addressing economic hardship among Americans, namely, American farmers. Policy pertaining to economic hardship is mental health policy. Economic hardship is linked to multiple poor mental health outcomes. In an analysis of nine waves (2001–2010) of nationally representative data from the Household, Income and Labour Dynamics in Australia Survey, involving 11,134 participants, economic hardship (deprivation and cash flow problems) was temporally associated with risk of mental health problems (Kiely et al. 2015). Data from the 2009 Swedish National Survey of Public Health (a randomly selected, representative national sample that included 23,153 men and 28,261 women ages 16–84 years) revealed that economic difficulties (inability to pay for ordinary bills, lack of cash reserves) were significantly associated with both women's and men's mental health indicators (psychological distress, severe anxiety, use of antidepressant medication) even after controlling for other variables such as educational level and employment status (Ahnquist and Wamala 2011).

In the United States, data from the 2016 and 2017 nationally representative National Surveys of Children's Health showed that family economic hardship is associated with each mental health condition examined, even after adjusting for covariates; hardship was associated with 84% increased odds of having an internalizing disorder and 53% increased odds of having externalizing (behavioral/conduct) problems (Assing-Murray and Lebrun-Harris 2020). Beyond economic hardship, income inequality and poverty have been linked to a wide array of negative mental health outcomes across the life span, with particularly deleterious and durable effects in children (Manseau 2015).

Similar findings have been documented for specific mental illnesses such as depression (Butterworth et al. 2009) among mothers in particular (Crosier et al. 2007), in especially vulnerable populations such as sexual minorities (Al-Ajlouni et al. 2020), and in the context of societal stressors such as the COVID-19 pandemic (Holingue et al. 2020; Kroska et al. 2020). At a societal level, extensive evidence has revealed that economic recessions and associated mediators such as unemployment, income decline, and unmanageable debts are significantly associated with poor mental well-being and increased rates of common mental disorders, substance use disorders, and suicidal behaviors (Frasquilho et al. 2016). Psychosocial interventions at the individual and family levels, as well as community-based interventions, have been suggested as a means of addressing economic hardship and thus mental health outcomes, although public policy interventions from the local to supranational levels are likely to have the greatest impact (Wahlbeck et al. 2017). The Farm Bills, across the generations, have reduced economic hardship among farmers and their families and have bolstered the economies of rural places and helped everyone in those communities, not just farmers, thus improving mental health and reducing risk of mental illnesses and substance use disorders.

As noted, in more recent decades, the Farm Bill has taken on the social determinant of health known as *food insecurity*, which is a condition at the individual or household level in which the availability of nutritionally adequate and safe foods or the ability to acquire such foods in socially acceptable ways is limited or uncertain, most often because of constrained financial resources. Although the original Farm Bill might not have directly targeted food security at a national level beyond farmers, later versions clearly have. Food insecurity, which in developed countries is nearly always driven by constrained financial resources, is clearly linked to depression and is likely linked to other specific mental illnesses, as well as one's general sense of well-being (Compton 2015). Longitudinal analyses suggest bidirectional relationships, with food insecurity increasing the risk of depressive symptoms or diagnosis and depression predicting food insecurity (Maynard et al. 2018).

In an analysis of data from 149 countries, food insecurity was shown to be associated, in a dose-response fashion, with poorer scores on mental health indices, even when controlling for diverse variables, including annual household income and employment status (Jones 2017). In a pooled meta-analysis involving data from 372,143 individual participants across 19 studies in 10 countries, a positive relationship was found between food insecurity and the risk of stress and depression, and food-insecure households living in North America had the highest risk of stress and anxiety (Pourmotabbed et al. 2020). Data from 5 years (2011–2015) of the National Health Interview Survey in the United States (N=124,343) revealed increasing odds of serious mental illnesses with increasing severity of food insecurity, and among individuals with such disorders, those with very low food security had about 2 times higher odds of not being able to afford mental health care and 25% lower odds of using mental health services than those who were food secure (Afulani et al. 2020). Clearly, food security is intimately linked to mental health, and measures that seek to address food security at the policy level, including the many food and nutrition assistance programs funded by the Farm Bill, have an impact on the nation's mental health. The Farm Bill is a mental health law, even though the original economists involved were not thinking about mental health and the connections between poverty, food security, and mental health at the time.

Since 2008, the Farm Bill has actually become a mental health law explicitly. The Farm and Ranch Stress Assistance Network (FRSAN) Program established a network that connects individuals engaged in farming, ranching, and other agriculture-related occupations to stress assistance programs. The network assists farmers in times of stress and can offer a conduit to improving behavioral health awareness, literacy, and outcomes for farmers and their families. This is partly driven by the known fact that farmers have higher suicide rates than the national average. The NY FarmNet program is an example of

FRSAN activity. It was initially created in 1986 as an initiative under a former dean of the Cornell College of Agriculture and Life Sciences, David Call. The program was designed originally as a safety net, with a toll-free phone number that farmers could call to gain access to a specialist to help alleviate stress, create emotional well-being, and address the mental health crisis among farm families that were then undergoing the farm crisis of the late 1980s. Over the program's evolution, Cornell recognized the linkage between the financial health of the farm and the emotional well-being of the farm family, and today, the program (funded by the New York State Department of Agriculture and Markets) sends a team of a financial consultant and a personal consultant to farms in distress. This synergistic approach to addressing the emotional or personal well-being needs of the farm family along with the seemingly inevitable underlying financial stress has assisted thousands of New York farmers over the years. NY FarmNet is part of the northeast FRSAN and has provided countless hours of training to mental health counselors (county and state personnel, primarily) in understanding the unique circumstances of farm families to better serve farmers in times of crisis, along with training agricultural business service providers to recognize stress in their clients and make appropriate referrals to NY Farm-Net for further assistance. More recently, in 2020–2021, the Coronavirus Food Assistance Program package for farmers contained $28 million for state block grants to work on mental health and stress-related issues for farmers.

As we have seen, the Farm Bill gets debated vigorously every few years, with different voices shaping adjustments and amendments to the bill over time. The voice of mental health has only recently been at the table, despite farm and food policy being mental health policy. What emerged from a national crisis, a dire crisis for farmers in particular, would become an evolving major economic policy, farming support policy, food security policy (and thus health policy), and, less apparently, a mental health policy. Its enactment initially required innovative and perhaps even untenable approaches, conceived by many politicians, agronomists, and economists such as Rexford Tugwell and others. They apparently did not have a mental health adviser then, but mental health should now have a place at the table. In addition to our being interested in the impact of the Farm Bill on economic viability and opportunity for farmers, as well as food security for all Americans, we should be interested in the ways in which farm and food policy in general might affect social determinants of mental health and, ultimately, mental health and mental illnesses in society.

References

Afulani PA, Coleman-Jensen A, Herman D: Food insecurity, mental health, and use of mental health services among nonelderly adults in the United States. J Hunger Environ Nutr 15(1):29–50, 2020

Ahnquist J, Wamala SP: Economic hardships in adulthood and mental health in Sweden: the Swedish National Public Health Survey 2009. BMC Public Health 11:788, 2011 21989478

Al-Ajlouni YA, Park SH, Safren SA, et al: High financial hardship and mental health burden among gay, bisexual and other men who have sex with men. J Gay Lesbian Ment Health 24(3):308–321, 2020 32884610

Assing-Murray E, Lebrun-Harris L: Associations between parent-reported family economic hardship and mental health conditions in U.S. children. J Child Poverty 26(2):191–214, 2020

Badger AJ: FDR: The First Hundred Days. New York, Hill & Wang, 2008

Butterworth P, Rodgers B, Windsor TD: Financial hardship, socio-economic position and depression: results from the PATH Through Life Survey. Soc Sci Med 69(2):229–237, 2009 19501441

Compton MT: Food insecurity, in The Social Determinants of Mental Health. Edited by Compton MT, Shim RS. Arlington, VA, American Psychiatric Publishing, 2015, pp 145–169

Conkin PK: The New Deal, 2nd Edition. Arlington Heights, IL, Harlan Davidson, 1987

Crosier T, Butterworth P, Rodgers B: Mental health problems among single and partnered mothers: the role of financial hardship and social support. Soc Psychiatry Psychiatr Epidemiol 42(1):6–13, 2007 17203237

Ducheneaux Z: American Rescue Plan socially disadvantaged farmer debt payments. Washington, DC, Farm Service Agency, U.S. Department of Agriculture, March 26, 2021. Available at: www.farmers.gov/blog/american-rescue-plan-socially-disadvantaged-farmer-debt-payments. Accessed February 1, 2022.

Farmers and Police Clash at Iowa Highway Blockade. Cincinnati Enquirer, August 25, 1932

Farmers Plan Protest Parade. Daily Argus-Leader (Sioux Falls, SD), September 22, 1932

Foster TB, Knop B, Bhaskar R: Access and eligibility for Supplemental Nutrition Assistance Program varies county by county. Suitland, MD, U.S. Census Bureau, February 2, 2021. Available at: www.census.gov/library/stories/2021/02/demographic-snapshot-not-everyone-eligible-for-food-assistance-program-receives-benefits.html. Accessed October 20, 2021.

Franklin Township in Somerset County, NJ, et al v Tugwell, Administrator, Resettlement Administration et al, 85 F2d 208 D. DC (1936). Available at: https://case.law.vlex.com/vid/85-f-2d-208-603169202. Accessed June 26, 2022.

Frasquilho D, Matos MG, Salonna F, et al: Mental health outcomes in times of economic recession: a systematic literature review. BMC Public Health 16:115, 2016 26847554

Georgia Farmers Dump Milk. Shreveport (LA) Times, September 27, 1932

Hall TG: Wilson and the food crisis: agricultural price control during World War I. Agricultural History 47:25–46, 1973

Hirth W: The gigantic farm debt. The Billings Times, December 32, 1932. Available at: www.shsmo.newspapers.com/image/580673840. Accessed December 4, 2020.

Holingue C, Kalb LG, Riehm KE, et al: Mental distress in the United States at the beginning of the COVID-19 pandemic. Am J Public Health 110(11):1628–1634, 2020 32941066

Imhoff D: Food Fight: The Citizen's Guide to the Next Food and Farm Bill. Berkeley, CA, Watershed Media, 2012

Jones AD: Food insecurity and mental health status: a global analysis of 149 countries. Am J Prev Med 53(2):264–273, 2017 28547747

Kiely KM, Leach LS, Olesen SC, et al: How financial hardship is associated with the onset of mental health problems over time. Soc Psychiatry Psychiatr Epidemiol 50(6):909–918, 2015 25683473

Kolb JH: Meeting the Farm Crisis. Chicago, IL, American Library Association, 1933

Kroska EB, Roche AI, Adamowicz JL, et al: Psychological flexibility in the context of COVID-19 adversity: associations with distress. J Contextual Behav Sci 18:28–33, 2020 32837889

Manseau MW: Economic inequality, poverty, and neighborhood deprivation, in The Social Determinants of Mental Health. Edited by Compton MT, Shim RS. Arlington, VA, American Psychiatric Publishing, 2015, pp 121–144

Maynard M, Andrade L, Packull-McCormick S, et al: Food insecurity and mental health among females in high-income countries. Int J Environ Res Public Health 15(7):1424, 2018 29986420

Montgomery DR: Soil erosion and agricultural sustainability. Proc Natl Acad Sci USA 104(33):13268–13272, 2007 17686990

Montgomery DR: Dirt: The Erosion of Civilizations, With a New Preface, 2nd Edition. Los Angeles, University of California Press, 2012

Namorato MV: Rexford G. Tugwell: A Biography. New York, Praeger, 1988

New York State College of Agriculture: Farm Economics, No 211. Ithaca, NY, Cornell University, December 1957. Available at: https://fraser.stlouisfed.org/files/docs/meltzer/peawar57.pdf. Accessed October 19, 2021.

Pigford v Glickman, civil action No 97-1978 (PLF) (1999). Available at: www.dm.usda.gov/pigford.pdf. Accessed June 19, 2022.

Pourmotabbed A, Moradi S, Babaei A, et al: Food insecurity and mental health: a systematic review and meta-analysis. Public Health Nutr 23(10):1778–1790, 2020 32174292

Rasmussen WD, Baker GL, Ward JS: A Short History of Agricultural Adjustment, 1933–1975 (Agriculture Information Bulletin No 391). Washington, DC, National Economic Analysis Division, Economic Research Service, U.S. Department of Agriculture. March 1976. Available at: https://naldc.nal.usda.gov/download/CAT87210025/PDF. Accessed October 22, 2021.

Roosevelt FD: Radio address on the National Democratic Platform From Albany, New York. Santa Barbara, CA, The American Presidency Project, July 30, 1932. Available at: www.presidency.ucsb.edu/documents/radio-address-the-national-democratic-platform-from-albany-new-york. Accessed June 26, 2022.

Tugwell RG: A Chronicle of Jeopardy, 1945–55. Chicago, IL, University of Chicago Press, 1955

Tugwell RG: The Art of Politics, as Practiced by Three Great Americans: Franklin Delano Roosevelt, Luis Munoz Marin, and Fiorello H. LaGuardia. Garden City, NJ, Doubleday, 1958

Tugwell RG: The Enlargement of the Presidency. Garden City, NJ, Doubleday, 1960

Tugwell RG: The Light of Other Days. Garden City, NJ, Doubleday, 1962

Tugwell RG: The Brains Trust. New York, Viking Press, 1968

U.S. Bureau of the Census: Historical Statistics of the United States, Colonial Times to 1957. Washington, DC, U.S. Department of Commerce, 1960, pp 122–123. Available at: f https://raser.stlouisfed.org/files/docs/publications/histstatus/hstat_1957_cen_1957.pdf. Accessed December 17, 2018.

U.S. Department of Agriculture: Key statistics and graphics. Washington, DC, Economic Research Service, 2021a. Available at: www.ers.usda.gov/topics/food-nutrition-assistance/food-security-in-the-us/key-statistics-graphics.aspx. Accessed October 20, 2021.

U.S. Department of Agriculture: Farming and farm income. Washington, DC, Economic Research Service, 2021b. Available at: www.ers.usda.gov/data-products/ag-and-food-statistics-charting-the-essentials/farming-and-farm-income. Accessed October 22, 2021.

Vilsack HJ: Just 0.1% of CFAP went to Black farmers. Ag Web Farm Journal, March 25, 2021. Available at: www.agweb.com/news/policy/politics/vilsack-just-01-cfap-went-black-farmers. Accessed October 22, 2021.

Wahlbeck K, Cresswell-Smith J, Haaramo P, et al: Interventions to mitigate the effects of poverty and inequality on mental health. Soc Psychiatry Psychiatr Epidemiol 52(5):505–514, 2017 28280872

White MM: Freedom Farmers: Agricultural Resistance and the Black Freedom Movement. Chapel Hill, University of North Carolina Press, 2018

3 | From Worker Exploitation to Union Solidarity

The National Labor Relations Act of 1935

Flávio Casoy, M.D.
Marc W. Manseau, M.D., M.P.H.

Long Fight for Better Pay and Better Working Conditions

Workers and bosses have been struggling against each other in America since the first British colonies. British colonial authorities had two purposes in promoting their North American colonies: the first was to reduce poverty in England, and the second was to transport idle and unproductive workers to the new world. These "workers" could then be exploited to establish the British colonial presence and enrich colonial leaders locally and in England. Twelve of the original colonists on the 1620 *Mayflower* were indentured and came unwillingly, and after 1630, fewer than half of colonists traveling to Massachusetts came for religious reasons (Isenberg 2017). It was common for wealthy families to own slaves and indentured servants, many of whom were abandoned children and were forced by English authorities to travel to the colonies (Murolo and Chitty 2001).

The first African slaves arrived in New Amsterdam (present-day New York) in 1626 and Boston in 1638. Colonial leaders often wrote to London asking for more indentured servants, and there was little recourse in the case of abuse or corruption. In fact, the enslavement of Native Americans and chattel slavery from Africa were the economic foundation of the 13 colonies, generating immeasurable suffering. The consequences of economic and political oppression of Native Americans, poor Europeans, and African Americans have dominated national politics since the start of the nation. Resistance to such oppression started immediately, and the first rebellion preceded even the first colonies. In 1526, 500 Spaniards and 100 enslaved Africans camped by the Pee Dee River in South Carolina. The slaves rebelled, killed most of the Spaniards, and escaped to nearby Native American settlements (Murolo and Chitty 2001). From the earliest times, the history of the United States has been marked by a continuous struggle between those who own farms, businesses, and factories and those whose work generates income for the owners.

From the beginning of the United States to the present day, numerous efforts have been made to control workers and make sure they remain divided and willing to work for less. State legislatures and courts tried throughout the colonial period, early republic, Civil War, and Reconstruction to prevent workers from forming organizations to demand better working conditions or more pay. However, by the late nineteenth century, tension was growing between a more progressive Congress that wished to provide relief to oppressed workers and more conservative courts that consistently ruled in favor of unfettered rights for business owners (Foner 1998).

Courts were the primary drivers of national labor policy through the nineteenth and early twentieth centuries. In the first half of the nineteenth century, courts often found that employees who worked together in negotiating with employers, even to raise wages, could be accused and tried in criminal courts (Leslie 2008). Courts often saw the mere threat to go on strike as a threat of violence and injury (Higgins et al. 2017). After the passage of the 1890 Sherman Antitrust Act—a great victory by reformists against monopolistic corporations—federal courts often misconstrued the broadly worded provisions of the Sherman Act to rule that collective action on the part of employees was anticompetitive and penalized workers with impossibly high fines (Boyer and Morais 1977).

A surge of progressive social legislation and investigative journalism—and a new social awakening—occurred around the turn of the nineteenth century. The contrast between a renewed aspiration for social justice and the underlying reality of child labor, gross exploitation of workers, and vast inequality in wealth grew untenable (Boyer and Morais 1977). It fueled the ongoing seesaw between a more progressive Congress and more conservative courts. Also, strikes against poor working conditions grew in number, and employers turned to increasingly violent methods to scare their employees into going back to work.

In response to the 1894 Pullman strike, a massive railroad strike that paralyzed rail travel in large parts of the country, President Grover Cleveland appointed a U.S. Strike Commission to investigate the causes. The commission found that if employers took "labor into consultation at proper times, much of the severity of strikes can be tempered and their numbers reduced" (United States Strike Commission 1895, p. LIV). The report resulted in the 1898 Erdman Act, which forbade firing employees for being in a union, mandated employers to work with unions representing employees, and created some mechanisms to resolve disputes (but the act applied only to trains that traveled between states). However, the Supreme Court found in *Adair v. United States* (1908) that provisions requiring railroad companies to recognize unions violated the Fifth Amendment rights of employers by infringing on their property rights without due process and that Congress did not have authority to pass such laws in their regulation of commerce powers (Higgins et al. 2017).

According to federal figures just after the turn of the twentieth century, approximately 2 million children around the country were required to work to supplement family incomes, with wages averaging less than $2 per week—equivalent to $55 in 2021 dollars. Almost one-half of working children were putting in 10 hours per day, 7 days per week. Fewer than 20% worked fewer than 8 hours per day. Women earned around $6 per week, or $165 in 2021. Two-thirds of working men earned less than $15 per week, or $413 in 2021. Almost half worked 12-hour days, 7 days per week. In 1914 alone, 35,000 workplace-related deaths occurred in the country's mines and factories. At the time, the federal Commission on Industrial Relations determined that half of those deaths were preventable. There were 700,000 nonfatal, but disabling, injuries that resulted in 4 weeks or more of inability to work (Commission on Industrial Relations 1915). Workers' homes were often little more than dormitories shared by dozens of people, where different shifts of workers shared the same beds while their fellow workers were on the job (Boyer and Morais 1977).

In September 1913, almost 11,000 workers of the Colorado Fuel and Iron Company (CFI) went on strike for an 8-hour day, a 10% pay increase, and better housing conditions. Similar to many companies at the time, CFI controlled almost every aspect of employees' lives. Employees lived on company land, in squalid and unsanitary conditions. The company deducted utilities and rent from their pay and forced them to shop for food and other necessities at the company store. Most workers quickly went into debt to the company, which meant they had to work longer and harder to pay off what they owed, creating a system akin to indentured servitude (Foner 1999).

CFI evicted the strikers from company housing and forced them and their families off company grounds; the striking workers settled to spend the winter in tent compounds, the largest of which was in Ludlow, Colorado. Concerned about the growing mass of angry, striking workers camped just outside company grounds, CFI hired gunmen from the Baldwin-Felts Detective Agency, who came into intermittent violent conflict with campers, prompting Colorado governor Elias Ammons to send the National Guard to restore order (at the encouragement of prominent CFI investor John D. Rockefeller). CFI repeatedly refused to meet and negotiate with the union, despite President Woodrow Wilson's attempt to broker an agreement. Tensions between the company, the union, and federal officials mounted, and violent skirmishes grew. On April 20, 1914, the Baldwin-Felts detectives and the Colorado National Guard sprayed the tents in the Ludlow camp with machine-gun fire, shredding many of the tents and killing the people inside. Drunken guardsmen later entered the camp and set fire to tents with oiled torches, shooting people as they stumbled away from the fires. Two women and 11 children were later found burned and asphyxiated by the smoke of their burning tent in a shallow, hand-dug bunker under one of the tents, where they had been hiding from the gunfire. A total of 21 workers were killed that day (Foner 1999). This atrocity became known as the Ludlow Massacre; it exemplifies the extreme risks workers had been taking to improve the deplorable working conditions that were the norm throughout the country's factories, mines, and ports.

Riding on the rage generated by the Ludlow Massacre, Congress responded to the Supreme Court's *Adair* and other decisions with passage of the 1914 Clayton Antitrust Act (Murolo and Chitty 2001). Although Congress could not pass legislation requiring employers to recognize unions because the Supreme Court had already ruled that to be unconstitutional, it amended the Sherman Act to significantly limit its use in suppressing labor activity. However, in *Duplex Printing Press Co v. Deering* (1921), the Supreme Court struck back with a very narrow read of the Clayton Act, which hobbled its efficacy in all but direct disputes between workers and employers, limiting activities such as boycotts of nonunion shops and solidarity strikes by other workers in the same industry (Leslie 2008).

Specter of Revolution

Industrial conflicts and strikes continued to mount throughout the 1910s and 1920s. Working people supported these strikes in increasing numbers and with growing determination. Businesses used their influence in state legislatures and with the courts to try to keep their employees from joining organizations and demanding better pay and better working conditions. They often resorted to hiring private detective agencies to use violence to intimidate their employees to prevent them from engaging in union activities. Just as it seemed that the social tensions between workers and their employers were reaching a bursting point, the stock market collapse in 1929 and ensuing economic depression rolled through the country, dramatically deepening the crisis. It was like a great natural disaster, but with no end from year to year between 1929 and 1933 and onward, getting worse and worse, more and more destructive. Instead of the calamitous brief destruction of a natural disaster, however, followed by waves of support from the Red Cross and other benevolent societies, millions of men and women faced catastrophe sitting and fretting alone at home. This was not just a global economic collapse, but an individual and deeply isolating collapse of self-worth and self-efficacy multiplied millions of times across the country. As a result, the class of workers fighting for union recognition swelled into the largest social movement the country had ever seen (Boyer and Morais 1977).

The National Unemployed Council was founded in 1930 in Chicago and quickly grew to have chapters in 46 states and almost every city and town in America. It explicitly opposed racial segregation and demanded relief for the unemployed, the hungry, and the homeless. It quickly became the primary national organization embodying the anger and despair of the millions thrown out of work during the Great Depression. A critical role it assumed was to prevent evictions. Hundreds of thousands of families were served with eviction notices for failure to pay rent or mortgages. In rural America, 1 million farmers lost their land to banks from 1929 to 1933, a problem the Agricultural Adjustment Act of 1933 would address. The Unemployed Council also mobilized thousands of unemployed workers to stand with striking workers and prevent bosses from hiring replacements and undercutting pay (Boyer and Morais 1977).

As the movement grew, many in power desperately tried to repress it. On March 6, 1930, at a national unemployment protest in Washington, D.C., police attacked hundreds of thousands of protesting workers from around the country with mounted officers and tear gas, including in front of the White House. Despite growing oppression, the Unemployed Councils continued to grow, diversify, and force relief bills through local government. Organizing blossomed around the country: in the South, the National Sharecroppers Union defied Jim Crow and united white and Black sharecroppers; across the Northeast and the Midwest, thousands of farmers blockaded roads in protest of the pricing of crops below cost. In March 1932, a march of unemployed workers in Dearborn, Michigan—named the

Ford Hunger March—ended with a police massacre of protestors (Boyer and Morais 1977).

In 1932, World War I veterans demanded immediate payment of a $50–$100 adjusted back pay bonus that had been approved in 1923. The movement began in April when Communist leaders of the Workers Ex-Servicemen's League demanded in a hearing of the House Ways and Means Committee that the bonus be paid immediately and not in 1945 when it was originally planned. For many, the amount of $50 or $100 meant the difference between keeping and losing a home. The Congressional committee refused, and the leaders called for a march on Washington. Given the growing despair, the response was much greater than anticipated, and with little planning or organization, veterans made their way to Washington from all over the country, often with their wives and children. On foot, on trains, in beaten-up old trucks, and on boats from as far as Alaska and Hawaii, groups converged on Washington hungry and tired, but determined. By June, under banners of "We fought for Democracy—Where is it?" and "Heroes in 1917—Bums in 1932," 25,000 people had camped across the Potomac in Anacostia Flats in caves, shacks, and huts or by just sleeping outside on the ground. Instead of respecting the rights of these veterans to meet and petition their representatives in Congress, the government decided they had to be disbursed. On July 28, alleging that the camps were full of criminals, President Herbert Hoover ordered the Army to disperse the veterans, which it did with cavalry and infantry. By midnight, the camp was in flames, and the veterans who had come to peacefully petition their Congress had been chased away from the city (Boyer and Morais 1977). Popular support was strongly with the veterans and other social movements, and in the election of 1932, Franklin D. Roosevelt soundly defeated Hoover (Murolo and Chitty 2001).

With Washington in new hands, Roosevelt and his allies in Congress immediately began to pass legislation to mobilize the federal government to provide relief for the millions stricken by the Depression. Foremost among these laws was the National Industrial Recovery Act (NIRA), which recognized in its Section 7A that workers had the right to bargain collectively through their own chosen representatives (Murolo and Chitty 2001). Although it would ultimately be deemed unconstitutional by the Supreme Court in 1935, NIRA opened the doors to mass collective organizing around the country. Millions of industrial workers along with whole new categories of white-collar, clerical, newspaper, and other service workers began to contemplate whether they could win better conditions through a union. Companies' reactions were swift, and they did everything in their power—including bribing local police, using violence, and intimidating workers—to prevent unions. In 1933, 900,000 workers went on strike for wage increases or union recognition. In 1934, 1.5 million workers struck in textile, coal, steel, automotive, meatpacking, beet sugar, and other industries all throughout the country. The pickets were violent, and many striking workers were killed. Yet the struggle persisted with increasing determination and ferocity (Boyer and Morais 1977).

It was in this massive social foment that 19-year-old Australian sailor Harry Bridges disembarked in San Francisco in 1920 (Figure 3–1). Having grown up in a staunchly pro-union family, he abandoned life as a sailor to work as a longshoreman in San Francisco. At the time, longshoremen in San Francisco were required to belong to a company union (a union formed and run by employers or their agents)—the Blue Book—because their prior union, the International Longshoremen's Association (ILA), lost a strike in 1919. When Bridges arrived in San Francisco, hiring for jobs was done daily, and workers had to "shape up," that is, humiliatingly line up before dawn and bribe company agents for jobs. When hired, they often had to work 24- to 36-hour shifts. It often took up to 6 days between shifts for workers to get rehired. The process was corrupt and degrading, and it left workers totally at the mercy of the whims of the hiring agents. Average pay was $10.45 per week ($141 in 2021 dollars). Bridges resisted this humiliation and worked as a "pirate" doing casual work around the docks and was then blacklisted after joining the ILA in 1924. He ultimately relented and joined the Blue Book and worked as a winch operator (Boyer and Morais 1977).

With the passage of NIRA in 1933, it became mandatory for shipping companies to negotiate with employees through any union they chose. Employers flouted the law despite orders by the regional federal labor board. By this time, Bridges had become influential on the docks through publishing a mimeograph pamphlet, the *Waterfront Worker* (Figure 3–2). He and several like-minded colleagues had been elected to the leadership of the newly constituted ILA that was organizing along the entire West Coast to force employers to follow the law and negotiate with the ILA. Bridges was elected chairman of the strike committee (Boyer and Morais 1977).

On May 9, 1934, longshoremen up and down the coast struck for union hiring halls, 30-hour work weeks, and pay increases. This strike effectively shut down the ports because longshoremen were required to load and unload the ships. On July 3, the police attacked the striking workers in San Francisco to make the strikers return to work and force open the port. The fighting lasted 2 days in "a hundred riots, big and little" (Boyer and Morais 1977, p. 285) with increasing reinforcement for both the police and for the striking workers from other unions. Police fired live ammunition while workers fought with bricks and clubs. On July 5, California governor Frank Merriam called out 2,000 soldiers of the National Guard, and Bridges decided to send the picketers home. Late in the evening of July 5, a call went out for a general strike in support of the striking longshoremen. The Painters' Union and Machin-

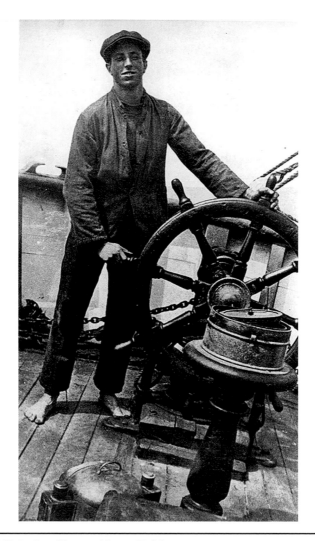

FIGURE 3–1.   Young Harry Bridges.

Source.   International Longshore and Warehouse Union Library and Archives, San Francisco, California. Photographer unknown. Available at: www.foundsf.org/index.php?title=File:Harry-Bridges-on-sailing-ship-young.jpg. Accessed May 11, 2022. Used with permission.

ists Union immediately supported the strike. On July 10, the Alameda Central Labor Council supported the strike, and on July 12, the powerful San Francisco and Oakland Teamsters gave its support. By the morning of July 16, industry in the Bay Area was at a complete standstill. Three thousand additional troops were sent to the city and, along with vigilantes, they destroyed union offices, bookstores, and newspaper presses, as well as other establish-

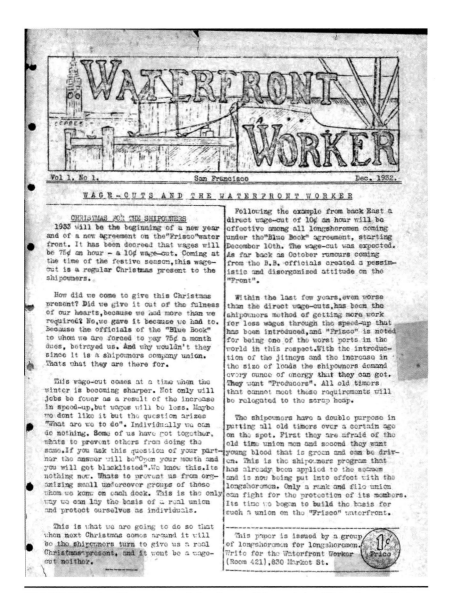

FIGURE 3–2. First page of the first edition of the *Waterfront Worker*.
Source. *Waterfront Worker* 1(1), 1932. International Longshore and Warehouse Union Library and Archives. Available at: http://archive.ilwu.org/wp-content/uploads/2015/04/WaterfrontWorker_1932-12-OCR.pdf. Accessed June 3, 2021. Used with permission.

ments seen to be progressive, yet the workers stayed home. The general strike ended on July 19, but National Guard and police troops did not again attack the striking longshoremen. The longshoreman strike ended on July

30, when the companies agreed to a union hiring hall with fair, rotational shift assignments; a 30-hour work week; and hourly pay. Bridges was elected president of the West Coast District of the ILA, and his leadership forever changed the dangerous, corrupt, and humiliating conditions at docks up and down the western United States (Boyer and Morais 1977).

The San Francisco General Strike was only one of many protracted, violent, and ultimately victorious labor struggles in 1934 and 1935. It was a product of enormous anger and thirst for organizing in the population, along with legal protections in NIRA. As labor battles mounted and more nonunionized industries were becoming organized, the Supreme Court threw out NIRA. Roosevelt and his allies in Congress were faced with a looming social revolution if they did not continue to provide substantive legislated relief. This chaotic, dangerous, and exciting dynamic set the stage for the country's most important legislation to protect workers' rights and dignity, the National Labor Relations Act (NLRA) of 1935, also known as the Wagner Act after Roosevelt's long-time supporter Robert Ferdinand Wagner (Murolo and Chitty 2001). Born in Prussia but having immigrated as a child to New York City, where his father worked as a janitor, Wagner was elected to the New York State Senate in 1909, where he served as chairman of the New York State Factory Investigating Commission, which looked into the 1911 Triangle Shirtwaist Factory fire, the deadliest industrial disaster in New York City (123 women and 23 men, mostly young factory workers, died in the fire). This investigation helped cement Wagner's dedication to protecting workers' rights and made him a leader of shepherding the later New Deal legislation through Congress after he was elected to the U.S. Senate in 1926 (U.S. Senate 2021).

National Labor Relations Act of 1935

The NLRA is the country's foundational policy on labor unions. Prior to it, there was no comprhensive policy guidance from the federal government, and there was a hodgepodge of incompatible, confusing rules from Congress, state legislatures, and federal courts. Only in response to massive social pressure were the architects of the New Deal able to create a more coherent national labor policy. The heart of the act is Section 7, which stipulates that "employees shall have the right to self-organization, to form, to join, or assist labor organizations, to bargain collectively through representatives of their own choosing, and to engage in other concerted activities for the purpose of collective bargaining or other mutual aid protection" (National Labor Relations Act of 1935).

In essence, the NLRA enshrines in law that workers are allowed to form unions. Another critical part of the act is the definition and banning of unfair labor practices by employers. Employers were banned from "interfering, restraining, or coercing" employees in any way that interferes in their exercising their right to form or join a union. It banned the formation of company unions similar to the Blue Book faced by Harry Bridges in San Francisco. The NLRA forbade employers from using hiring, firing, promotions, and other employment decisions to discriminate against employees because of union activity or for testifying before the National Labor Relations Board (NLRB). The NLRA also deemed employers' refusing to negotiate in good faith with unions or other duly established representatives of their employees an unfair labor practice.

The NLRA established the NLRB to administer the act and interpret unfair labor practices. The five members of the NLRB are appointed by the president and confirmed by the Senate. A general counsel, also appointed by the president and confirmed by the Senate, serves to supervise NLRB attorneys and the regional offices. The NLRB can delegate authority to regional boards and administrative law judges.

When a group of workers wishes to form a union via the NLRA, the first step is to determine the bargaining unit. The bargaining unit is ultimately determined in a hearing by the NLRB with inputs from both workers and employers. It is the "unit appropriate to assure to employees the fullest freedom in exercising the rights guaranteed" in the act. A bargaining unit can be geographical and/or based on the type of work or educational background. A bargaining unit cannot include both professional and nonprofessional employees unless a majority votes for such a unit. In the act, a professional employee is defined as performing work that is "predominantly intellectual and varied in character as opposed to routine mental, manual, mechanical, or physical work." Units cannot include security guards whose job is to protect employer property or enforce rules against other employees. The act also does not apply to farm workers, public sector workers, independent contractors, domestic workers, or any worker whose job falls under the Railway Labor Act of 1926 (National Labor Relations Act of 1935).

In order to begin the process under the NLRA, the employees who wish to form a union need 30% of employees who form the bargaining unit to sign a petition to the NLRB for a union election. If the employer does not recognize the representative of the union or if there is a dispute about the nature of the bargaining unit, then a hearing must take place. Provided the NLRB finds that the bargaining unit is appropriate and that the employees who are petitioning to form a union are appropriate under the NLRA, then it sponsors a secret ballot election in which all the members of the proposed bargaining unit are invited to vote whether to form a union. Going from the initial petition to the election can take years, and the findings of the

NLRB are heavily influenced by the party affiliations and political ideologies of its members. Once an election is held, should a majority of the unit vote in favor of the union, the employer must negotiate with the workers' chosen representative. Decisions by regional boards can be appealed to the NLRB in Washington, D.C., or to a federal appeals court (National Labor Relations Act of 1935).

In addition to the 1935 Wagner Act, Congress passed the Fair Labor Standards Act in 1938. The Fair Labor Standards Act establishes a minimum wage, overtime pay eligibility, record-keeping standards, and child labor standards. It has been amended numerous times since its passage, and courts have weighed in repeatedly to clarify how to apply the language (Fair Labor Standards Act of 1938). Such clarification is important in the context of the Wagner Act discussion because the Wagner Act does not create a floor of working conditions that employers must meet; it provides only a mechanism for workers to bargain collectively.

Even with these two landmark pieces of legislation, progress was not steady. About a decade later, over President Harry S. Truman's veto, a more conservative Congress passed the Taft-Hartley Act of 1947. Taft-Hartley shifted the federal government's position from being explicitly pro-union to making unions harder to form. Taft-Hartley amended the original Wagner Act to create a category of certain prohibited practices by unions. These included prohibitions against engaging in solidarity strikes with employees of other companies that are nonunion, as well as strikes to force employers to fire specific employees for not belonging to the union (Leslie 2008).

Taft-Hartley also amended the original Wagner Act to include in the centrally important Section 7 the right to *not* join a union. This outlawed closed shop and union shop workplaces in the United States. Prior to Taft-Hartley, employers that had a unionized workplace could hire only union members or individuals who agreed to immediately join the union. Union members who violated union rules and were expelled from the union would lose their jobs (Murolo and Chitty 2001). Since Taft-Hartley, two categories of union workplaces have existed in the United States: *agency shops* and *open shops* (Boyer and Morais 1977).

In agency shops, workers who are not members of the union are required to pay an *agency* fee to cover the cost of the union's negotiating the contract and for any representational needs the worker may have. Under a union contract, even workers who are not members of the union have the right to be represented by the union in any disputes they may have with the employer; agency fees cover these costs. They are generally less than union dues because nonunion workers generally do not participate in the social and organizational events union members enjoy. Union members often donate to a separate political action fund for unions' political activities.

In open shops, workers who are not members of the union are not required to pay agency fees even though they remain entitled to the contract negotiated by the union and representation in case they get in trouble at work. Since the passage of Taft-Hartley, 28 states have passed laws that ban agency shops; these laws are also (somewhat euphemistically) called *right to work laws*. Union membership in these states is much lower because unions are required to provide services to so-called "freeloaders" and often have fewer resources for organizing and negotiating better contracts.

Because of Taft-Hartley and other anti-union measures, the rate of unionization in the United States has been steadily dropping from its post–World War II peak. In 2020, 10.8% of the workforce was in a union, down from 20.1% in 1983, when systematic data collection on union membership began. The fall has been most precipitous in states that enacted laws against agency shops. Private sector unionization has fallen especially precipitously; workers in the public sector now have a fivefold higher unionization rate than workers in the private sector: 34.8% and 6.3%, respectively (U.S. Bureau of Labor Statistics, 2021).

Today, about half the unionized workforce is covered by the Wagner Act and subsequent amendments. State and local public employees have their union rights defined by state laws. Federal unions are governed by the 1978 Federal Labor Relations Act. In a much-debated 5–4 opinion, the Supreme Court handed down a decision in *Janus v. American Federation of State, County, and Municipal Employees Council 31* (2018) that limits the power of unions. In the *Janus* decision, the court ruled that because public sector unions negotiate with elected officials to obtain more favorable contracts for their members, the core contract negotiating work can be considered political lobbying and therefore political speech. The Supreme Court ruled that for this reason, paying an agency fee is a violation of nonunion workers' First Amendment rights and that therefore all public sector workplaces must be open shops and not agency shops. This creates a large incentive for people to "free load," that is, to receive the benefits of having a union without paying the dues that unions need to maintain these benefits. The full effect of this decision has yet to be determined, but public sector unions are preparing for a drop in their membership and revenue as their ability to represent members shrinks.

Getting Under the Skin: How the Right to Organize Results in Better Mental Health

The medical and public health literature has paid little attention to the direct connection between union membership and health or mental health outcomes. However, using logistic regression and propensity score matching to a nonunion control population, one study did show that union membership is associated with better self-reported health (Reynolds and Brady 2012). This study also showed that the relationship between union membership and better health is explained mostly through higher wages and therefore incomes among union members, although income differences do not entirely explain this relationship among all subpopulations in the study (e.g., low-education workers). Although more research is necessary to elucidate the direct relationship between union membership and mental health outcomes, unions affect multiple conditions of work that have been demonstrated to influence mental health.

First, unions increase wages, increase income, and decrease poverty rates among both unionized and nonunionized employees within industries and labor markets. After the passage of NIRA in 1933 and subsequently the NLRA in 1935, significant growth of the unionized workforce occurred throughout the country. The early industrial unions transformed dangerous industrial and mining jobs into a safer and steady path to the middle class for millions of workers. Today, unions transform low-wage jobs in hospitality, health care, janitorial, and other service sectors into positions with living wages and better benefits, lifting those workers out of poverty. On average, union workers earn 13% more than workers with similar education, experience, and occupations who are not in a union. In service occupations such as food and janitorial services, union workers may earn 56% more in wages (and 87% more in total compensation) than their nonunion peers. Even for nonunion workers, when union density is high, wages across the board tend to go up because unions create an upward pressure on wages and sometimes can negotiate for better wages sector-wide, even for workers who are not their members (Bivens et al. 2017).

In addition to increasing negotiating power for workers, unions increase wages because union workers tend to be more aware of their rights and have more avenues to fight back if employers engage in violations of local or federal laws. This prevents wage theft, overtime violations, off-the-clock violations, meal break violations, illegal deductions, and other violations. Nonunion employees are much more likely to take home less than what they are entitled to, which results in a significantly higher risk of poverty (Cooper and Kroeger 2017).

Unions also help reduce family poverty. In addition to having better pay, union workers are more likely to have health insurance that covers families and dependents, protecting them from overwhelming debts and bankruptcies related to medical illness. This protects workers from falling behind on rent or other expenses, reducing the risk of homelessness and other bad outcomes. Through pension programs and other retirement programs, union workers have much better retirement security than nonunion workers. This helps protect workers from poverty once they retire. Retirement income can help ensure continued housing not only for the retired worker but also for adult children and grandchildren (Bivens et al. 2017).

Low income and poverty are significant social determinants of physical health outcomes, including, but not limited to, adult mortality (Kondo et al. 2009) and life expectancy (Wilkinson 1992), infant mortality and other birth outcomes (Metcalfe et al. 2011), cardiovascular disease (Clark et al. 2009), and self-reported physical well-being (Kondo et al. 2009). Since the 1970s, numerous psychiatric and social epidemiological studies have found that people living in poverty are also at increased risk for various poor mental health outcomes, including depression, anxiety disorders, traumatic experiences, suicide, and substance use (Kingston 2013; Li et al. 2011; Sareen et al. 2011). Additionally, people who live in poverty have significant difficulty accessing preventive and therapeutic health care services (Hodgkinson et al. 2017). Children are at particularly high risk for an array of poor mental health outcomes associated with poverty, including lower school achievement, higher rates of depression and anxiety, and worse cognitive and behavioral outcomes (McLoyd 1998; Yoshikawa et al. 2012). As union membership has dropped over the latter decades of the twentieth century and the early twenty-first century, childhood poverty has increased, creating what has been called a *juvenilization* of poverty in the United States. For instance, in 2012, almost 40% of children in the United States were poor or near poor, and in 2013, a majority of U.S. public school students were low income and eligible for free- and reduced-lunch programs (DeNavas-Walt et al. 2013).

People of racial and ethnic minoritized backgrounds in the United States have lower incomes and lower family wealth and are more likely to live in poverty; as such, they are more likely to experience adverse physical and mental health effects of economic deprivation (Hanks et al. 2018). In addition, women earn less than men for the same work (Barroso and Brown 2021). However, union membership has increasingly become a force against these gender- and racial- and ethnic-based economic disparities (Bivens et al. 2017). Two-thirds of union workers are women and/or people of color (Economic Policy Institute 2021). In this way, the labor movement has at least partially overcome its checkered history when it comes to fighting racism and sexism. Particularly prior to the 1930s, the American Federation of Labor was a strong advocate for segregation and racist immigration laws. However, following the Unemployed Councils of the early 1930s and the organization of the Congress of Industrial Organizations in 1935, the newly formed industrial labor unions increasingly battled racial segregation and sexism. Although regressive attitudes regarding race and sex unfortunately persist in some union locals even today, the labor movement as a whole has kept a continued focus on organizing the lowest-income sectors of society and has, as a result, been a significant avenue for women and racially minoritized people to join the middle class. For instance, today, a higher percentage of Black and Hispanic workers are unionized than white workers (Bivens et al. 2017). Furthermore, recent research has suggested that union membership may lessen attitudes of racial resentment and increase support among white workers for policies that benefit people of color, thereby countering increasing racist and white supremacist attitudes among some sectors of the white working class (Frymer and Grumbach 2021).

In increasing wages and incomes, unions have historically also been a major driving force—even the main driver—of reducing social and economic inequality in the United States. Unions decrease inequality because they tend to give a larger wage boost to low- and middle-income occupations than to high-income occupations. Black and Hispanic workers have greater improvements than white workers, in large part because they start at lower pay compared with white workers. Unions also tend to enter industries with more low- and middle-income workers, resulting in a boost in those wages. Declines in union representations explains one-third of the rise of wage inequality among men and one-fifth of increasing inequality among women from 1973 to 2007 (Bivens et al. 2017). From the early twentieth century through the early twenty-first century, union membership rates have correlated strongly with income inequality in the United States (Figure 3–3), with inequality dropping as union membership rose through the 1950s and with income disparities rising precipitously again as union membership ebbed, a trend that accelerated after the 1970s (Kimball and Mishel 2015).

Inequality has increased precipitously since 1980 because wages for workers have stagnated even as worker productivity has steadily increased. From 1979 to 2015, hourly pay has grown 0.3% per year, or 9.9% in total. If pay increases had kept up with rising productivity, as they did in the decades prior to 1979, pay would have risen by 63.8% (Bivens et al. 2017). This expected rise did not happen, however, because ever-larger shares of the economic pie have been going to the highest earners, driving an accelerating income inequality. As a result, between 1979 and 2005, the top 1% of income earners in the United States had an income growth of 150%, whereas the lowest 40% of earners saw largely stagnant wages (Gould 2013); in 2012, almost a quarter of total income in the United States went to the top 5% of earners, whereas only 3% went to the bottom 20% (DeNavas-Walt et al. 2013). Working people use unions and their power in numbers to secure a fairer share of the wealth their work creates. As unions decline, employers can more easily take and keep that wealth for themselves (Bivens et al. 2017).

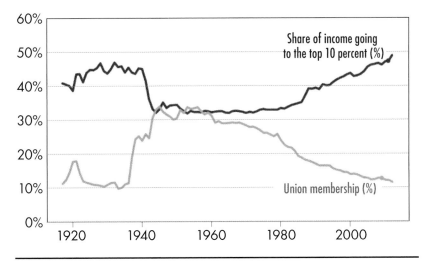

FIGURE 3–3. Union membership rates and income inequality, 1917–2013.
Source. Re-created with data from Kimball and Mishel 2015.

This rising inequality in the United States has negative implications for population health and mental health. Significant evidence shows that inequality above and beyond poverty contributes to overall worse health outcomes, including increased infant mortality (Metcalfe et al. 2011) and lower life expectancy (Kondo et al. 2009; Wilkinson 1992), among other outcomes. Population-level income inequality has also been associated with poor mental health outcomes at multiple levels of analysis (e.g., national, state, county) and for multiple types of outcomes, including adult depression rates (Messias et al. 2011; Muramatsu 2003; Pabayo et al. 2014), drug overdose death rates (Nandi et al. 2006), and an index of childhood well-being that includes mental health variables (Pickett and Wilkinson 2007).

Unions also provide a powerful mechanism for workers to improve multiple noneconomic conditions of work. In addition to negotiating wages, hours, safety enhancements, benefits, and so forth, they can also negotiate for formal mechanisms to resolve workplace conflicts and help level the power difference between employees and managers (Cooper and Kroeger 2017). Union contracts generally also allow employees who find themselves in high-stress situations, such as being victims of workplace accidents, being subject to disciplinary hearings, and being victims of harassment, to bring a union steward or staff member with them to meetings with managers or company executives; this protects the employee from feeling isolated or intimidated (Bivens et al. 2017). Contracts also often mandate the presence of a union representative in injury and fatality investigations, ensuring that they are thorough. As a result, unions have led to vastly safer work-places throughout the twentieth century and beyond (Centers for Disease Control and Prevention 1999). In addition to lowering risk of injury and death, improved workplace conditions and better safety measures have the potential to improve mental well-being among workers (Russo et al. 2019).

Feeling unheard, powerless, or disrespected at work is an experience that likely all employees have experienced at some point in their working lives, and this has the potential to negatively affect mental health. In fact, a higher sense of control and decision-making autonomy in a job has been associated with better mental health and well-being (Bentley et al. 2015). When a union is present in a workplace, a mechanism exists to address systemic conditions that leave workers feeling powerless. With a union, employees can come together and have a legally recognized voice in their workplace. Unions can also include in contracts specific benefits to protect workers' mental health. For example, as of June 2017, Texas state firefighters have had greater workers' compensation coverage for workers diagnosed with line-of-duty-related PTSD (Bivens et al. 2017).

Last, but certainly not least, unions have been instrumental in fighting for and protecting the progress gained from other policy advances such as the Social Security Act and the Civil Rights Act that are also discussed in this book. Across the twentieth century, unions have been a primary political voice for working people. Just as corporations and business interest groups hire lobbyists to represent their interests in Washington, D.C., unions can help push for policies that affect all workers, such as protecting social security, health and safety laws, minimum wage laws, and health care access laws (such as the 2010 Patient Protection and Affordable Care Act). In fact, research shows that union membership—especially among less educated workers, who are generally less likely to be politically engaged—is associated with being more politically active in ways that range from voting to organizing protests. As such, union membership is associated with general civic engagement and volunteerism, suggesting that union activity specifically increases political capital (which leads to greater power) (Kerrissey and Schofer 2013). As union strength has waned in the United States in recent years, social protections that had been taken for granted, such as overtime pay and retirement pensions, have come under attack. A significant decline has also occurred in the real value of the minimum wage, which is lower today than it was in 1970. Even with diminished power, unions remain a driving force behind critical legislation that can improve inequality. For example, the fight for a $15/hour minimum wage that was started by the Service Employees International Union in New York City and Chicago has spread nationally and—short of a federal minimum wage increase—has already resulted in improved wages for countless fast food and other service workers. Unions are pushing for other legislated rights such as guaranteed paid sick leave, predictable scheduling, and universal prekindergarten around the country (Bivens et al. 2017).

Dusk or a New Dawn: Labor Faces an Uncertain Future

The influence of labor unions has been waning for decades in the United States, which has brought in its wake rising levels of inequality (almost unprecedented), stagnant wages and a shrinking middle class, increasingly exploitative working conditions, and, recently, political instability. Although large decreases in labor union membership are not the only cause of these complex economic trends (other causes include, but are not limited to, technological changes and globalization), many prominent economists agree that the decline of unions has been a major driving force (Krugman 2021). Attention on the population-wide mental health harms that these economic trends have caused is increasing. For instance, one groundbreaking study showed that between 1999 and 2013, middle-age, non-college-educated (i.e., working class) white people in the United States experienced a decrease in life expectancy, representing the only population-level reversal following decades of progress in life expectancy in the industrialized world until the coronavirus SARS-CoV-2 disease (COVID-19) pandemic (Case and Deaton 2015). Furthermore, this population-level loss of life expectancy was explained primarily by increases in mental health–related problems: drug overdoses, suicides, and deaths from alcohol-related liver disease.

In order to reverse these economic trends and set the American people's mental health status back in a positive direction, it is essential that participation in organized labor increase in the United States. However, numerous significant barriers to this happening exist. Although the NLRA protected the rights of workers to organize without sanctions or intimidation from employers, provisions in the law have often gone unenforced under both Democratic and Republican administrations, especially since the 1970s, making it often cheaper and easier for employers to risk violating the law than to comply with it (Bouie 2021). And even when the law is enforced, it is often only after lengthy and drawn-out NLRB proceedings, resulting in mild sanctions such as employer agreements to not violate the law in the future or to pay back lost wages for workers (but not punitive fines for the employers). Furthermore, current federal law requires unions to organize one workplace at a time (i.e., not an entire company or industry) and allows employers to severely restrict access to workplaces for union organizers and to flood employees with anti-union messages in the workplaces, including through mandatory anti-union meetings (Scheiber 2021). In June 2021, the Supreme Court decided in the 6–3 *Cedar Point Nursery v. Hassid* (2021) decision that a California law allowing union organizers to enter an employer's property is unconstitutional, making it even more difficult for union organizers to talk to workers (Howe 2021).

Recent structural changes to the U.S. economy have added other barriers to unionization and have further decreased the rate of union membership. These include the rise of contract and long-term freelance work—including the "gig" economy, such as ride sharing services—that is often indistinguishable from other types of employment in any way other than name. This allows companies to label individuals who would otherwise be employees as private contractors, who are then exempt from most of the rights and protections of labor and employment law, including the right to organize and join a union (Kim 2021). In addition, as manufacturing jobs have declined in the United States, a large rise in low-wage work in the services industries (e.g., the food service industry) has occurred (Collins 2016), leading to many disempowered workers who are vulnerable and have little recourse to employer abuses such as last-minute work schedule changes (creating uncertainty similar to the shape-up process faced by Harry Bridges on the San Francisco docks in the 1920s and 1930s) and wage theft (Bivens et al. 2017).

Finally, political and legal threats to labor organizing in the United States have been increasing. The *Janus v. AFSCME* Supreme Court decision came down at the same time that states were increasingly passing right to work laws, both of which are certain to decrease union membership in the years ahead, and President Donald J. Trump appointed people openly hostile to unions to the NLRB, including its general counsel. However, the U.S. labor movement has some reason for hope on the horizon. President Joseph R. Biden has taken an early strong prolabor stance, and in moves unprecedented for any sitting president since Franklin D. Roosevelt, he fired the Trump-appointed NLRB general counsel before the end of the counsel's term and gave an unequivocally pro-union speech during a campaign to organize an Amazon facility in Alabama (Bouie 2021). The U.S. House of Representatives also passed the Protecting the Right to Organize Act, which would strengthen the right to organize in numerous ways, including, but not limited to, strengthening penalties on employers who violate labor law, banning anti-union employer practices such as mandatory anti-union meetings, limiting the scope of right to work laws, and allowing many employees currently classified as contract workers to unionize (Fandos 2021). If it is passed by the Senate (President Biden has said he would sign it), the Protecting the Right to Organize Act would be the most significant expansion of labor rights since the NLRA. The bill passed in the House of Representatives by a vote of 225 to 206 on March 9, 2021. At the writing of this chapter, the bill has advanced to the Senate, although its future is uncertain because it would require universal Democratic support and 10 Republican crossover votes to pass in case of a filibuster.

The labor movement in the United States has been far from perfect. Especially early on, the movement and its achievements left out many women as well as Black and brown people. The NLRA often lacked the enforcement teeth necessary to actually protect workers, even prior to its subsequent erosion by state and federal legislation and court decisions, and the NLRB was too open to political ideology and interference. The legal and organizational structure of organized labor became calcified and unable to flexibly and quickly respond to the dynamics of a rapidly changing global economy. However, labor organizing has been and remains the most powerful tool that workers have at their disposal to match the might of their employers and industry. Business owners and employers often have vast resources and powerful political connections on their side, but workers have each other in large numbers and the ability to withhold the work that generates wealth. However, in order to continue to leverage the power of labor organizing, we will need a *new labor* that corrects deficiencies in the legal protections for unions, addresses historical inequities within the labor movement, allows unions to more flexibly adjust to current and future economic realities, and, most importantly, increases rates of union membership. And because labor organizing gets at the heart of power differentials within society, this would have the added advantage of strengthening our democracy and making it more possible to enact policies that would improve many of the social determinants of mental health. The CFI strikers in the early twentieth century and the San Francisco dock workers in the 1930s alike recognized that they were fighting for much more than better pay and working conditions—they were fighting for a freer and more equal society—and the United States still needs labor organizing to serve this function a century later. Although policy makers and politicians ultimately had to pass the law, the true heroes, like Harry Bridges, rose up as regular workers, inspiring any and all of us to stand up not only for justice in wages, safety, and benefits but also for a right to mental health.

References

Adair v United States, 208 US 161 (1908)

Barroso A, Brown A: Gender pay gap in U.S. held steady in 2020. Washington, DC, Pew Research Center, 2021. Available at: www.pewresearch.org/fact-tank/2021/05/25/gender-pay-gap-facts. Accessed June 17, 2021.

Bentley RJ, Kavanagh A, Krnjacki L, LaMontagne AD: A longitudinal analysis of changes in job control and mental health. Am J Epidemiol 182(4):328–334, 2015 26138706

Bivens J, Engdahl L, Gould E, et al: How today's unions help working people: giving workers the power to improve their jobs and unrig the economy. Washington, DC, Economic Policy Institute, August 24, 2017. Available at: www.epi.org/publication/how-todays-unions-help-working-people-giving-workers-the-power-to-improve-their-jobs-and-unrig-the-economy/. Accessed June 16, 2021.

Bouie J: Biden is saying things Amazon doesn't want to hear. The New York Times, March 2, 2021. Available at: www.sltrib.com/opinion/commentary/2021/03/11/jamelle-bouie-biden-is/. Accessed February 3, 2022.

Boyer RO, Morais HM: Labor's Untold Story: The Adventure Story of the Battles, Betrayals, and Victories of American Working Men and Women. New York, United Electrical, Machine, and Radio Workers of America, 1977

Case A, Deaton A: Rising morbidity and mortality in midlife among white non-Hispanic Americans in the 21st century. Proc Natl Acad Sci USA 112(49):15078–15083, 2015 26575631

Cedar Point Nursery v Hassid, 594 US __ (2021)

Centers for Disease Control and Prevention: Improvements in workplace safety—United States, 1900–1999. MMWR Morb Mortal Wkly Rep 48(22):461–469, 1999 10428100

Clark AM, DesMeules M, Luo W, et al: Socioeconomic status and cardiovascular disease: risks and implications for care. Nat Rev Cardiol 6(11):712–722, 2009 19770848

Collins M: Where have all the good paying jobs gone? IndustryWeek, March 4, 2016. Available at: www.industryweek.com/the-economy/public-policy/article/22007276/where-have-all-the-good-paying-jobs-gone. Accessed June 17, 2021.

Commission on Industrial Relations: Final Report and Testimony Submitted to Congress by the Commission on Industrial Relations Created by the Act of August 23, 1912. Washington, DC, U.S. Congress, 1915

Cooper D, Kroeger T: Employers steal billions from workers' paychecks each year: survey data show millions of workers are paid less than the minimum wage, at significant cost to taxpayers and state economies. Washington, DC, Economic Policy Institute, May 10, 2017. Available at: www.epi.org/publication/employers-steal-billions-from-workers-paychecks-each-year-survey-data-show-millions-of-workers-are-paid-less-than-the-minimum-wage-at-significant-cost-to-taxpayers-and-state-economies. Accessed June 6, 2021.

DeNavas-Walt C, Proctor BD, Smith JC: Income, Poverty, and Health Insurance Coverage in the United States: 2012. Washington, DC, U.S. Census Bureau, 2013

Duplex Printing Press Co v Deering, 254 US 443 (1921)

Economic Policy Institute: Who are today's union workers? Fact Sheet. Washington, DC, Economic Policy Institute, April 21, 2021. Available at: www.epi.org/publication/who-are-todays-union-workers/. Accessed June 17, 2021.

Fair Labor Standards Act of 1938, Pub. L. No. 75-718, sec. 203, 52 Stat. 1060–1070.

Fandos N: House passes labor rights expansion, but Senate chances are slim. The New York Times, March 9, 2021. Available at: www.nytimes.com/2021/03/09/us/politics/house-labor-rights-bill.html. Accessed February 3, 2022.

Foner PS: History of the Labor Movement in the United States, Vol 2: From the Founding of the A.F. of L. to the Emergence of American Imperialism. New York, International Publishers, 1998

Foner PS: History of the Labor Movement in the United States, Vol 5: The AFL in the Progressive Era. New York, International Publishers, 1999

Frymer P, Grumbach JM: Labor unions and white racial politics. Am J Pol Sci 65(1):225–240, 2021

Gould E: The top one percent take home 20% of America's income. Washington, DC, Economic Policy Institute, July 18, 2013. Available at: www.epi.org/publication/top-1-earners-home-20-americas-income. Accessed June 4, 2021.

Hanks A, Solomon D, Weller CE: Systematic inequality: how America's structural racism helped create the Black-white wealth gap. Washington, DC, Center for American Progress, February 21, 2018. Available at: www.americanprogress.org/issues/race/reports/2018/02/21/447051/systematic-inequality. Accessed June 4, 2021.

Higgins JE, Deady PE, Torres JJ, et al; ABA Committee of Development of the Law Under National Labor Relations Act; ABA Section of Labor and Employment Law: The Board, the Courts, and the National Labor Relations Act. Arlington, VA, Bloomberg BNA, 2017

Hodgkinson S, Godoy L, Beers LS, et al: Improving mental health access for low-income children and families in the primary care setting. Pediatrics 139(1):e20151175, 2017 27965378

Howe A: Court holds that regulation guaranteeing union access to employees is unconstitutional. SCOTUSblog, June 23, 2021. Available at: www.scotusblog.com/2021/06/court-holds-that-regulation-guaranteeing-union-access-to-employees-is-unconstitutional. Accessed June 23, 2021.

Isenberg N: White Trash: The 400-Year Untold History of Class in America. New York, Penguin Books, 2017

Janus v American Federation of State, County, and Municipal Employees Council 31, 138 S Ct 2448, 201 L. Ed. 2d 924 (2018)

Kerrissey J, Schofer E: Union membership and political participation in the United States. Soc Forces 91:895–928, 2013

Kim ET: Freelancers shouldn't have "horror stories." The New York Times, March 25, 2021 Available at: www.nytimes.com/2021/03/25/opinion/pro-act-biden-labor.html?. Accessed February 3, 2022.

Kimball W, Mishel L: Unions' decline and the rise of the top 10%'s share of income. Washington, DC, Economic Policy Institute, 2015. Available at: www.epi.org/publication/unions-decline-and-the-rise-of-the-top-10-percents-share-of-income. Accessed June 4, 2021.

Kingston S: Economic adversity and depressive symptoms in mothers: do marital status and perceived social support matter? Am J Community Psychol 52(3–4):359–366, 2013 24122088

Kondo N, Sembajwe G, Kawachi I, et al: Income inequality, mortality, and self rated health: meta-analysis of multilevel studies. BMJ 339:b4471, 2009 19903981

Krugman P: America needs to empower workers again. The New York Times, April 12, 2021. Available at: www.nytimes.com/2021/04/12/opinion/us-unions-amazon.html. Accessed February 3, 2022.

Leslie DL: Labor Law in a Nutshell, 5th Edition. St. Paul, MN, Thomson West, 2008

Li Z, Page A, Martin G, et al: Attributable risk of psychiatric and socio-economic factors for suicide from individual-level, population-based studies: a systematic review. Soc Sci Med 72(4):608–616, 2011 21211874

McLoyd VC: Socioeconomic disadvantage and child development. Am Psychol 53(2):185–204, 1998 9491747

Messias E, Eaton WW, Grooms AN: Economic grand rounds: income inequality and depression prevalence across the United States: an ecological study. Psychiatr Serv 62(7):710–712, 2011 21724781

Metcalfe A, Lail P, Ghali WA, et al: The association between neighbourhoods and adverse birth outcomes: a systematic review and meta-analysis of multi-level studies. Paediatr Perinat Epidemiol 25(3):236–245, 2011 21470263

Muramatsu N: County-level income inequality and depression among older Americans. Health Serv Res 38(6 Pt 2):1863–1883, 2003 14727801

Murolo P, Chitty AB: From the Folks Who Brought You the Weekend: A Short, Illustrated History of Labor in the United States. New York, New Press, 2001

Nandi A, Galea S, Ahern J, et al: What explains the association between neighborhood-level income inequality and the risk of fatal overdose in New York City? Soc Sci Med 63(3):662–674, 2006 16597478

National Labor Relations Act of 1935, 29 U.S.C. § 151 et seq.

Pabayo R, Kawachi I, Gilman SE: Income inequality among American states and the incidence of major depression. J Epidemiol Community Health 68(2):110–115, 2014 24064745

Pickett KE, Wilkinson RG: Child wellbeing and income inequality in rich societies: ecological cross sectional study. BMJ 335(7629):1080–1086, 2007 18024483

Reynolds M, Brady D: Union membership and self-rated health in the United States. Soc Forces 90:1023–1049, 2012

Russo M, Lucifora C, Pucciarelli F, et al: Work hazards and workers' mental health: an investigation based on the fifth European Working Conditions Survey. Med Lav 110(2):115–129, 2019 30990473

Sareen J, Afifi TO, McMillan KA, et al: Relationship between household income and mental disorders: findings from a population-based longitudinal study. Arch Gen Psychiatry 68(4):419–427, 2011 21464366

Scheiber N: Biden may be the most pro-labor president ever; that may not save unions. The New York Times, March 25, 2021. Available at: www.nytimes.com/2021/03/25/business/economy/joe-biden-unions.html. Accessed February 3, 2022.

United States Strike Commission: Report on the Chicago Strike of June-July 1894. Washington, DC. Government Printing Office, 1895. Available at: http://moses.law.umn.edu/darrow/documents/Report_on_the_Chicago_Strike_of_June_July_1894_appendices.pdf. Accessed June 13, 2022.

U.S. Bureau of Labor Statistics: Economic news release: union members summary. Washington, DC, US. Bureau of Labor Statistics, 2021. Available at: www.bls.gov/news.release/union2.nr0.htm. Accessed February 3, 2022.

U.S. Senate: Robert Wagner: a featured biography. Washington, DC, U.S. Senate, 2021. Available at: www.senate.gov/senators/FeaturedBios/Featured_Bio_Wagner.htm. Accessed June 16, 2021.

Wilkinson RG: Income distribution and life expectancy. BMJ 304(6820):165–168, 1992 1637372

Yoshikawa H, Aber JL, Beardslee WR: The effects of poverty on the mental, emotional, and behavioral health of children and youth: implications for prevention. Am Psychol 67(4):272–284, 2012 22583341

4 | A Stay Against Financial Catastrophe

The Social Security Act of 1935

Caroline L. Bersak, Esq.
Matthew Wolfe, B.A., M.A., M.Phil.

"Do Something as Soon as Possible": Depression Era Crisis of Livelihood and Care

In 1933, a few months into his presidency, President Franklin Delano Roosevelt received a letter from a Mrs. M.A. Zoller of Beaumont, Texas, requesting assistance for her 81-year-old mother. Her mother, Zoller wrote, was "helpless, suffering from Sugar Diabetes, which has affected her mind," leaving her "to be cared for in the same manner as an infant." Her savings exhausted and falling into debt, Zoller implored the president to "do something...as soon as possible" (Hiltzik 2011, p. 238).

At the height of the Great Depression, many people caring for elderly loved ones in the United States found themselves in similarly desperate straits. Such widespread anxiety about the welfare of elderly people, however, was a relatively modern phenomenon. Until this time, providing for those who needed assistance—including elderly and poor people and persons with disabilities—had generally been left to families and to private charitable groups. No large-scale federal programs to provide citizens with income or other forms of support and few state and local options existed. In the early twentieth century, the patchwork system of family support, local charities, poorhouses, and poor farms (county- or town-run residences where impoverished elderly and disabled people lived) began to fail. Urbanization, spurred on by the Industrial Revolution, pushed many workers out of rural areas toward cities, leaving fewer people to tend to family members left behind. Around the same time, people began living longer—between 1910 and 1930, advances in public health increased average life expectancy by 10 years—leading to significant growth in the elderly population. However, retirement benefits and pensions from employers were still relatively rare, causing a conspicuous gap in income and care.

During the Roaring Twenties, the booming U.S. economy served to paper over growing income inequality and a burgeoning credit bubble. However, the stock market crash of 1929 and the subsequent Great Depression pushed an already fragile system to its breaking point. Between 1930 and 1933, unemployment increased, disastrously, from around 10% to almost 30%. People who managed to keep their jobs faced pay cuts. Foreclosures, repossessions, and evictions increased rapidly, as did homelessness. Many breadwinners left their families and took to the road in search of work. A 1933 *New York Times* article described a "nomad horde" of more than a million people "wandering up and down the country" ("1,250,000 Homeless Reported in Nation" 1933). Familial ties to those needing care became ever more strained.

Children, meanwhile, frequently found themselves separated from impoverished parents. Wanda Bridgeforth, who was a child in Chicago during the Depression, recalled her father, an African American man with a degree in chemistry, breaking down over the humiliation and anxiety of unemployment. Her mother was ultimately forced to find work as a live-in domestic worker. Beginning in grade school, Bridgeforth was boarded and sent to live with a succession of relatives and strangers (Ellis 2008).

The Progressive movement responded to this crisis by championing old-age pensions, as well as mothers' aid and widows' pensions, which consisted of cash payments for widowed mothers that enabled them to care for children at home. Although many states adopted one or both assistance programs, their administration was inconsistent and unreliable. Often, a program would be passed into law but receive no funding. By the early 1930s, for example, a majority of states had enacted mothers' aid programs, but only a quarter were funded (Piven and Cloward 2012). The needy, then, remained heavily reliant on private charitable organizations for aid, but with the unprecedented demand, these organizations soon began to falter. As the crisis facing vulnerable populations deepened, the federal government fell under increasing pressure to provide for the country's needy.

Witnessing the Crisis: Frances Perkins and the Origins of Social Security

Frances Perkins was a trailblazer in several realms. Not only was she the first woman to hold a number of powerful positions in state and federal government, but she was also the driving force behind many of the most progressive policies of the New Deal, including, most famously, the Social Security Act of 1935 (Figure 4–1). Born in 1880 and raised in Massachusetts and Maine, Perkins would soon shed her family's New England conservatism to become one of the country's most influential reformers. While attending Mount Holyoke College in western Massachusetts, Perkins fell under the wing of Florence Kelley, then executive secretary of the National Consumer League, a progressive group dedicated to labor protections and reform. After college, while teaching at Ferry Hall, a women's college in Chicago, Perkins became friendly with many of the city's influential progressives and soon began working at one of the nation's oldest settlement houses, Hull House, which provided a variety of social services in poor, urban areas, often serving immigrant communities (Downey 2009).

Increasingly passionate about social work, Perkins took a job in Philadelphia investigating and protecting immigrant women who were forced into sexual slavery and other coercive labor. After a brief stint studying economics at the University of Pennsylvania's Wharton School of Business, Perkins took a fellowship at Columbia University. In New York City, she was offered a job heading the local office of the National Consumer League, still run by her mentor, Florence Kelley. This position allowed her to make powerful contacts in Tammany Hall, the city's Democratic headquarters, and in Albany.

Many of Perkins's social welfare commitments were inspired by personal experiences. In 1911, she bore firsthand witness to the Triangle Shirtwaist Factory fire in New York City, one of the nation's worst industrial tragedies, in which 146 people lost their lives. Before the blaze, the factory's stairwell doors were locked to prevent workers—mostly young immigrant women and teenagers—from stealing or taking unauthorized breaks. Perkins, who lived only blocks from the factory, witnessed workers jumping to their death to flee the inferno. Shortly after the tragedy, Perkins was recommended by former president Theodore Roosevelt to lead the new Committee on Safety, which set about to reform unsafe labor conditions (Sprague 2014). A few years later, Perkins had her first child, spurring her to accept a new position as executive secretary of the Maternity Center Association, which sought to improve dismal maternal and infant health outcomes, especially among low-income and immigrant populations (Downey 2009).

Perkins's connections to politicians and policy makers helped her star rise, and she soon established herself as a national expert on issues of employment and labor. In 1918, Perkins's friend Al Smith was elected governor of New York. He gave Perkins her first political appointment, making her a member of the New York State Industrial Commission, which oversaw conditions in factories throughout the state. Perkins was the first woman to sit on the commission, at a time when women still lacked the right to vote. Finally, in 1928, newly elected governor Franklin Delano Roosevelt appointed Perkins as industrial commissioner for the state of New York, putting her in charge of one of the state's largest administrative agencies. As the head of New York's labor and industrial agency, Perkins found herself in a particularly influential position just as the Great Depression began wreaking havoc on the country's economy. Early in her tenure, she pushed Roosevelt to adopt state unemployment insurance and old-age pension plans, traveling to England to study their dole program. In January 1930, Perkins made national headlines by disputing President Herbert Hoover's claim that employment was on the rise, criticizing the statistics put out by the Department of Labor as inaccurate ("Disputes Hoover on 'gains' of nation" 1930).

In 1933, as Roosevelt took office as president, Perkins joined his administration as secretary of labor, making her the first woman in U.S. history to hold a cabinet position, at a moment when labor policy was more relevant than ever. Before accepting the appointment, Perkins made clear to Roosevelt that she intended to fight for a number of groundbreaking programs, including unemployment insurance payments, old-age pensions, health insurance, workers' compensation, and labor protections. Although Roosevelt was initially reluctant, Perkins set about convincing him that such programs were necessary, advisable, and possible. In 1934, Roosevelt was sufficiently persuaded that he made Perkins the chairwoman of his Committee on Economic Security, established to study and propose solutions for economic and social security at a national level. This commission would ultimately make the recommendations and proposals that became the basis for the Social Security Act of 1935.

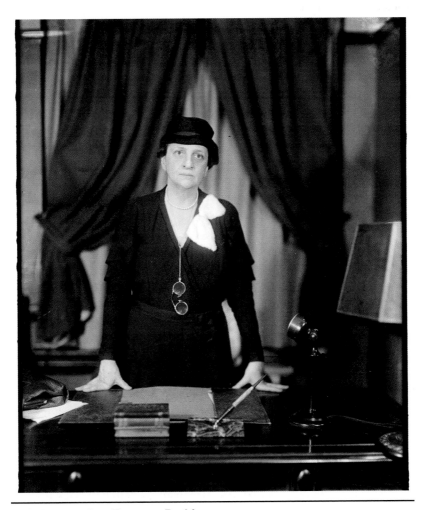

FIGURE 4–1.   Frances Perkins.

Frances Perkins was the first woman appointed to a U.S. presidential cabinet position and remains the longest-serving U.S. secretary of labor.

Source.   Library of Congress, Prints & Photographs Division, photograph by Harris & Ewing, LC-DIG-hec-21647. Available at: www.loc.gov/item/2016862692. Accessed February 3, 2022.

Again, Perkins's personal experiences may have informed her policy proposals. Her husband struggled with a serious mental illness, most likely bipolar disorder, and spent the majority of his adult life unable to work, residing in institutions. (On the day the first Social Security Act was signed into law by Roosevelt, Perkins had to race back to New York because her husband had absconded from a hospital.) Throughout her adult life, Perkins was also responsible for supporting and caring for her elderly mother. Saddled with the

costs of paying for her husband's ongoing care and providing for her mother
and daughter, Perkins struggled financially and was forced to rely on the gen-
erosity of wealthy friends to meet her family's needs (Downey 2009).

A Wealth of Plans:
Congress Considers Solutions

Even as the Great Depression worsened in the early 1930s, President
Hoover failed to acknowledge the depth of the crisis. Opposed to government intervention, Hoover encouraged charities and localities to bear the
burdens of the Depression, refusing calls for relief laws and vetoing a bill
that would have provided for federal public works and employment programs. Local relief programs, however, were overwhelmed. In 1933, *The
New York Times* reported that the number of meals and nights of lodgings
provided to the homeless by relief organizations had more than quadrupled
since the Depression's onset ("Aid to Homeless" 1933).

Roosevelt was elected in November 1932 with a strong mandate to
change strategies. However, although he had campaigned on expanding
federal assistance, he had offered few details of his plans. When he took office, he set about translating his ideas into policy. In May 1933, the Federal
Emergency Relief Administration, a precursor to many of the programs
created by the Social Security Act, was created, allocating $500 million for
states to help the unemployed. Other early Roosevelt administration legislation focused on creating jobs, such as the Civilian Conservation Corps,
Civil Works Administration, and Public Works Administration. Many others outside the administration had ideas, too, and countless activists offered
Roosevelt their own plans for improving economic security. "When I got
to my office as Secretary of Labor in 1933," Frances Perkins explained, "I
found on [the] desk over 2,000 plans" (Perkins 1962). Perkins was struck by
how many of these plans included forms of social insurance.

One of the more popular proposals came from Senator Huey Long of
Louisiana. With the slogan "Every Man a King," Long's 1934 Share Our
Wealth plan sought to mitigate the massive economic inequality he thought
to be a primary cause of the Depression. His plan included proposals to
place a $50 million cap on private individual wealth; to limit annual incomes
and inheritances to $1 million and $5 million, respectively; and to guaran-
tee every family an annual income of at least $2,000 (approximately $39,466
in 2021 dollars, adjusted for inflation). Long's plan also included old-age
pensions for those older than age 60 and a 30-hour work week, with 4 weeks
of vacation. A network of Share Our Wealth clubs sprang up throughout

the country; by 1935, there were more than 27,000 chapters, with more than 7 million members (McElvaine 2000).

Dr. Francis E. Townsend, a physician living in Southern California, proposed his own plan, focused on providing for seniors and elderly people. Dr. Townsend was inspired to action after observing elderly women picking through garbage cans for food during the Depression ("Doctor's Plan of Guaranteed Aid Started It" 1985). First proposed in 1933, the Townsend Plan was simple: government pensions of $200 per month (approximately $3,977 in 2021 dollars) for all retired citizens older than age 60, paid for by issuing bonds and enacting a federal sales tax. Pensioners would be required to take an oath to spend the entire $200 each month within the United States and to forego any work and other forms of private income to further stimulate the economy (Foote 1934). Despite its popularity among the public, the plan was criticized for being economically infeasible, with one organization claiming it would cost one-half of the entire national income ("Pension Proposal Called Fantastic" 1934).

In 1934, seeking his own plan, Roosevelt created the President's Committee on Economic Security (CES), charged with studying problems related to the economic security of individuals, with Frances Perkins as chairwoman. Working at a remarkable pace, the CES provided its findings and recommendations to Roosevelt within 6 months. Its report, issued just before Christmas, would serve as a comprehensive road map for what would ultimately become the Social Security Act. "The one almost all-embracing measure of security is an assured income," the report stated in its introduction. "A program of economic security, as we vision it, must have as its primary aim the assurance of an adequate income to each human being in childhood, youth, middle age, or old age—in sickness or in health" (President's Committee on Economic Security 1935). The report's major recommendations and provisions included the following:

- *Employment assurance*, described as "the stimulation of private employment and the provision of public employment for those able-bodied workers whom industry cannot employ at a given time"
- *Unemployment compensation*, to be administered by states, with guidance from the federal government and funded by a payroll tax
- *Old-age security*, a contributory system of old-age annuities to benefit younger workers on their retirement along with noncontributory pensions for those now old with no means of support
- *Security for children*, recommending federal grants to states for expenditures to support children and young families "without a breadwinner" and including aid for the care of "crippled and handicapped" children

- *Risks arising out of ill health*, recommending a preventive public health program to be administered by states and localities with funding and assistance from the federal government

In January 1935, Roosevelt sent the proposed legislation to both houses of Congress, urging that it be enacted without delay (President's Committee on Economic Security 1935). The resulting bill, called the Economic Security Act, was not without controversy. Shortly after its introduction, a *New York Times* article claimed that the CES had ignored the advice and recommendations of experts, who counseled that unemployment compensation should be a national program rather than a joint federal-state plan and that the Old-Age Insurance program would be rendered insolvent (Stark 1935b). Congressional hearings on the bill seemed to create more confusion. Feeling that the omnibus bill was too large and complex, many congressional representatives favored breaking up the bill into its various component programs for individual consideration (Stark 1935a). Business and industry interests opposed the new taxes imposed by the unemployment insurance and old-age pension programs ("The Security Bill" 1935). The unemployment insurance provisions were also criticized by those who thought they would reward idleness or laziness. "The unemployment insurance idea was full of hazards for many people," said Perkins, "and particularly for the politicians, who tended to take the old-fashioned view that there was something wrong with people who were unemployed, and that they ought to bear the burden of their own sins" (Perkins 1962).

By March, *The New York Times* was predicting that the omnibus bill would fail and that the only measures likely to be enacted were the assistance for needy elderly people and child welfare (Stark 1935a). However, despite the opposition, the Social Security Act, as it was renamed during congressional consideration, eventually passed both houses of Congress. After its passage, *The New York Times* noted that "since more than forty million people would share ultimately in the benefits provided by the measure, to vote against it was, as some members remarked privately, 'to invite political suicide'" ("Security Bill Challenged" 1935).

Social Security Act of 1935

Most Americans today are familiar with Social Security, often associating it with a federal program of retirement benefits. But this retirement program was only a small part of the 1935 Social Security Act. Moreover, many of the programs run by today's Social Security Administration were not part of the original 1935 law but were added through further legislation over time. The 1935 act created a framework for various economic, social, and health programs with a special focus on "needy" individuals: children, the unemployed, and elderly people. The foundation for these programs laid by the 1935 Social Security Act still, in large part, underpins most of the welfare and poverty relief programs that remain in effect in the United States today.

Consisting of 11 titles, the act created a set of relief programs that generally fell within four main categories: a federal old-age pension for retired workers; a federal-state unemployment insurance program; federal funding for state programs providing financial assistance to certain categories of needy people; and services to children, mothers, and individuals with disabilities (Social Security Act of 1935).

Federal Old-Age Benefits

The Social Security retirement benefits with which many people are now familiar were largely established by Title II of the act, which created a federal program of "old-age benefits": monthly payments to qualified individuals age 65 and older based on their work history (Figure 4–2). Individual work histories and earnings would be tracked beginning in 1937 (leading to the invention of the social security number). Among other eligibility requirements, individuals qualified for these benefits by having worked in at least 5 calendar years between 1937 and their 65th birthday and having earned a minimum of $2,000 during that time. Payments to individuals were to begin in 1942, although later legislation accelerated that to 1940. The amount of the monthly payment was calculated individually on the basis of each person's earnings from employment after 1936, up to a maximum payment of $85 per month (approximately $1,652 in 2021). The monthly payment would be reduced if a person continued to work after age 65.

Importantly, workers in many types of employment were explicitly excluded from participating in Social Security's old-age benefits program. The act specified that earnings from agricultural labor; domestic service; serving as officers and crew of U.S. or foreign ships; government employment; and employment by religious, charitable, and other not-for-profit institutions would not count toward creating eligibility for the program. This meant that huge numbers of American workers—in particular, people of color and many others who worked in physically demanding and relatively low paying jobs—would not qualify for federal old-age benefits.

Unemployment Compensation

The Social Security Act also created a framework for state programs to provide financial assistance to the unemployed, clearly a significant concern at

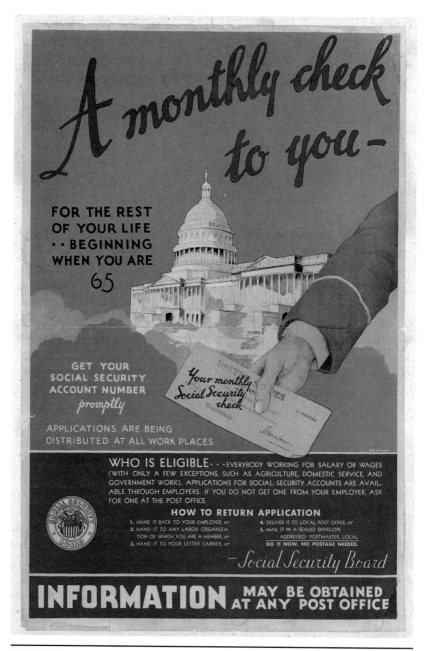

FIGURE 4–2.   Social Security Administration promotional poster distributed to familiarize Americans with the new retirement benefits.

Source. Washington, DC, Social Security Board, 1935. Available at: www.loc.gov/resource/ppmsca.07216. Accessed: July 5, 2022.

the time. Titles III and IX of the act authorized federal payments to states whose unemployment compensation programs met minimal administrative standards. This model gave states significant freedom in designing and implementing unemployment compensation plans, including setting most eligibility requirements and benefit amounts. Unlike with other programs, the 1935 act did not set guidelines or limits on the amount of benefits payable to individuals as unemployment compensation. The act appropriated a set amount of federal dollars toward the administrative costs of the programs and established a federal Unemployment Trust Fund and a tax on most employers to cover the costs of payments to unemployed individuals. As with Title II's old-age benefits, workers in certain types of employment were excluded from the unemployment compensation program. This meant that a significant portion of American workers could not receive unemployment benefits if they lost their jobs, with a disproportionate impact on African American workers based on the exclusion of domestic and agricultural laborers (Rodems and Shaefer 2016).

State Programs for Aid to the Needy

In addition to establishing a system of benefits for many workers on retirement or in the event of unemployment, various titles of the act created additional programs to assist specific categories of the needy. Title I authorized a joint federal-state program for assistance to "aged needy individuals." Ostensibly, this program would provide some minimal financial assistance to people who did not qualify for the federal old-age benefits described above. Participating states would be required to provide payments to eligible individuals, focusing first on those age 70 and older and then expanding to include eligible individuals 65 and older by 1940. A similar program that provided assistance to "needy individuals who are blind" was included in Title X of the act. Under these programs, the federal government would make payments to states that adopted plans for financial aid to needy elderly and blind individuals if those plans met the minimal standards laid out in the act. A third program included in Title IV of the Social Security Act authorized federal funds to partially reimburse states for payments under approved programs for aid to "needy dependent children." The act defined a dependent child as one who was younger than age 16, lived with certain specified relatives, and was "deprived of" support or care from one or both parents because of death, absence, or physical or mental incapacity.

The Social Security Act did not require states to adopt these programs and merely provided for federal cost sharing if states did enact approved programs. The act gave states significant flexibility in designing and implementing plans with respect to eligibility, benefit amounts, and more. But the levels of federal reimbursement to states for such programs were limited to a paltry amount of monthly benefits for such individuals. For programs aiding elderly and blind people, federal funds would cover half of the amount states spent on payments to eligible individuals, but only up to a maximum of $30 per month per individual (roughly equal to $583 in 2021). For assistance to dependent children, federal funds would cover just one-third of state payments and only up to a maximum of $18 per month for the first dependent child in a household (worth approximately $350 in 2021) plus an additional $12 per month for any additional dependent children in the household. Although the act did not prohibit states from giving more generous amounts to their needy citizens, any payments over the maximums set in the act would come entirely out of state or local budgets.

Federal Funding for Services

The 1935 Social Security Act also allocated federal funding for various kinds of services, aside from direct financial assistance to individuals. Title V authorized federal funding, with particular focus on rural areas and areas in severe economic distress, for 1) services promoting the health of mothers and children; 2) medical and other services for "crippled children" or children with conditions that could cause "crippling"; 3) services for the protection and care of children who were homeless, dependent, neglected, or at risk of becoming delinquent; and 4) vocational rehabilitation for individuals with physical disabilities to promote return to civil employment. Title VI authorized federal funding to assist states with establishing and maintaining public health services and provided funding to the Federal Public Health Service to work with states on the investigation of diseases and enhancements to sanitation.

An Even Newer Deal: The Evolution of Social Security and the Public Safety Net

The Social Security Act of 1935 laid the foundation for the United States' largest financial assistance and welfare programs, nearly all of which are still operating today. Many of today's safety net benefits were not included in the original 1935 legislation, which has been amended dozens of times since 1935. Many of these amendments expanded or added programs and benefits, although in more recent years, amendments have tended to restrict eligibility. Some of the more significant changes to the Social Security Act are discussed in the following subsections, with the exception of the 1965 amendments that established the Medicaid and Medicare health insurance programs, which are beyond the scope of this chapter.

Creation of the Federal Old-Age, Survivors, and Disability Insurance Programs

Numerous amendments and additions over the past nine decades have expanded the original program of federal old-age benefits for retired workers into the sprawling amalgam of benefits programs currently operated by the Social Security Administration. The first major changes came in 1939, just a few years after the original act was passed and before payments under some of the programs had even begun. Whereas the 1935 act created a program for payments to only the individual retired worker, the 1939 amendments allowed for monthly payments to certain dependents or surviving family members of a worker, signaling a focus on ensuring financial security of entire families. Eligible family members included the wife and minor children of a retired worker and, in the event of a worker's premature death, his widow, minor children, and/or parents (Social Security Act Amendments of 1939). Gender-based distinctions in benefits eligibility, particularly for dependents and survivors of workers, were included in Social Security legislation for decades, relying on increasingly outdated assumptions that men were the sole or primary income earners in families. The 1939 Social Security Act Amendments also modified how workers qualified for retirement benefits, specifically using the language and concept of "insurance." Taking into account these changes, the 1939 act called the program Federal Old-Age and Survivors Insurance Benefits. In 1950 and again in 1954, amendments to the Social Security Act extended eligibility for old-age and survivors benefits to many categories of workers who had previously been excluded, including many domestic and agricultural workers; certain self-employed persons; some government workers; and employees of religious, nonprofit, and charitable organizations under certain circumstances (Social Security Act Amendments of 1950; Social Security Amendments of 1954). The 1983 amendments expanded eligibility to even more categories, although some workers, including employees of many state and local government entities, were still excluded (Social Security Amendments of 1983).

One of the most significant changes to the Old-Age and Survivors Insurance program occurred in 1956, when it became the Old-Age, Survivors, and Disability Insurance (OASDI) program, after Congress authorized eligibility for benefits based on disability, rather than just on a worker's death or retirement (Social Security Amendments of 1956). *Disability* was given a strict definition based on a person's long-term or permanent inability to earn money through work because of a physical or mental impairment. Workers who were insured (by meeting specific requirements related to length of work history and amount of earnings) could qualify for monthly payments if they became disabled between ages 50 and 65. (By 1960, Congress expanded eligibility for disability benefits to insured workers of any age, not just those 50 and older.) The 1956 amendments also added monthly benefits for disabled children of insured retirees or insured deceased workers; children could receive these benefits through adulthood if their disability began before age 18 and would continue.

Finally, the act was amended a number of times to change how benefits under the OASDI program were calculated and, in some circumstances, to allow for higher monthly payments. In response to growing concern about the financial stability of Social Security, a comprehensive reform bill was passed in 1983. In addition to making changes in how the program was funded, the 1983 amendments increased the age at which a worker could retire and receive full benefits, with the increase to be phased in slowly over a number of years (Social Security Amendments of 1983).

Evolution of Programs for the Needy

Following the passage of the Social Security Act in 1935, states were largely left on their own to create and implement programs for aid to the needy (blind and elderly people, dependent children). The 1939 Social Security Act Amendments added the requirement that states take into account other income and resources of people applying for such assistance when determining need, formally making these means-tested benefits. In 1950, before the addition of disability insurance benefits, Congress added Title XIV to the Social Security Act, appropriating federal funds to reimburse states for payments to needy individuals who are "permanently and totally disabled," creating a program that functioned like the existing assistance programs for needy, elderly, and blind people (Social Security Act Amendments of 1950).

By far the largest change to these public assistance programs came in 1972 when Congress created the Supplemental Security Income (SSI) program (Title XVI of the Social Security Act), a federal program for monthly payments to individuals who are older than age 65, blind, or disabled and who have little or no other income and few assets (Social Security Amendments of 1972). In contrast to Social Security's OASDI program, individuals did not need to be "insured" on the basis of work history to be eligible for SSI benefits; people who had never worked at all could receive benefits under this program if they met the other eligibility requirements. The definition of disability was the same as the one used for Social Security's Disability Insurance program. Monthly payments under the SSI program were (and still are) quite low—below the federal poverty level—and are reduced if the recipient has other income or receives other types of in-kind support (such as living somewhere rent free). In 1974, when SSI payments first began, the maximum federal benefit amount for an individual under the SSI program was $130 per month (about $733 in 2021 dollars). In 2021, the maximum federal benefit amount was $794 per month for an individual or $1,191 per month for married couples in which both spouses are eligible (Social Security Administration 2021b).

At the same time the SSI program was enacted, Congress repealed the titles of the Social Security Act (as amended) that authorized the joint federal-state programs for aid to needy elderly, blind, and disabled people (Titles I, X, and XIV) but continued to allow for federal payments to states to cover rehabilitation and other services to needy elderly, disabled, or blind individuals.

Creation of Welfare as We Know It

The Aid to Dependent Children (ADC) program underwent myriad changes and amendments, but the program laid out in the 1935 Social Security Act is still largely the foundation of the current Temporary Assistance to Needy Families (TANF) program, or what is commonly referred to as *welfare*. Other than adjustments for inflation, the benefit amounts for this type of assistance have not increased significantly in the past nine decades. For example, in 2021, the maximum assistance amount for one child receiving TANF benefits in New York City was $183 per month in cash payments plus $277 to go toward rent or housing costs (paid only if the recipient family can show a rent or other housing payment obligation of at least that amount) (New York Codes, Rules, and Regulations 2020).

As with other forms of assistance from the 1935 act, early amendments to ADC tended to expand the program, whereas more recent amendments have tended to restrict or limit benefits. In 1939, Congress slightly increased the allowable rates of federal reimbursement for state expenses and expanded the definition of *dependent child* to include a child up to 18 years old if that child regularly attended school (Social Security Act Amendments of 1939). A relatively significant expansion occurred in the 1950 Social Security Act Amendments, with new legislation allowing payments to be made for the needs of an adult caretaker relative in the home, rather than just for the dependent children, and allowing some federal reimbursement of state payments for certain medical care of dependent children and the caretaker relative. In 1961, Congress allowed states to provide assistance to families that were needy because of a parent's unemployment in addition to a parent's absence, death, or incapacity (An Act to Amend Title IV of the Social Security Act to Authorize Federal Financial Participation in Aid to Dependent Children of Unemployed Parents, and for Other Purposes of 1961). Reflecting the expansion of payments and services, Congress in 1962 formally changed the program name from Aid to Dependent Children to Aid to Families with Dependent Children (AFDC; Public Welfare Amendments of 1962).

Later that same decade, Congress began to pass legislation that seemed to be aimed at reducing the number of recipients of these types of benefits. In 1967, Congress required state programs to provide child welfare and other services to AFDC families, including services to assist people receiving AFDC benefits in entering the work force and services to reduce out-of-wedlock births. The 1967 Social Security Amendments created a formal Work Incentive Program to help place AFDC recipients into employment and work training, allowing states to determine which recipients should participate in work programs (Social Security Amendments of 1967). Subsequent amendments added more specific requirements as to who must participate in work training programs. In 1996, the Personal Responsibility and Work Opportunity Reconciliation Act signed by President Bill Clinton repealed the AFDC program and replaced it with the TANF program. Despite Clinton's campaign pledge to "end welfare as we know it," the TANF program kept in place the joint federal-state program model, with many of the same eligibility rules, but added stricter work requirements. Under the TANF program, significant changes were made to the way federal funding was given to states: states would now receive block grants and were given broad leeway in determining how to spend the grants. Perhaps most significantly, the Personal Responsibility and Work Opportunity Reconciliation Act added a time limit for this type of assistance. With few exceptions, states were prohibited from using federal funds to provide assistance to families in which an adult had received TANF benefits for more than 60 months cumulatively throughout their life (Personal Responsibility and Work Opportunity Reconciliation Act of 1996).

Impact of Increasing Income for Millions of Americans on Mental Health

The Social Security Act of 1935 laid the foundation for nearly all of the United States' income security and safety net programs. The sheer number and variety of programs the act spawned complicate any comprehensive discussion of the legislation and its effects. Moreover, even within certain programs, such as TANF and unemployment benefits, states have freedom to implement vastly different rules and benefits, yielding more than 50 different plans for each program. However, what unites the programs of the Social Security Act and their progeny is that nearly all of them provide recipients direct payments of cash. The TANF program, which grew out of the 1935 act's ADC program, provides subsistence support to 1.1 million families with children annually as of 2017 (Becker 2018). The original programs for state plans to aid needy, elderly, and blind people have been combined and expanded into today's federal SSI program, which provides subsistence income to more than 8 million elderly, blind, and disabled individuals each year (Social Security Administration 2018). The federal-state unemployment insurance program included in the original Social Security Act still operates more or less as originally designed. The old-age pensions have grown into Social Security's OASDI program, which provides qualified workers and their families with some level of retirement pension, life insurance, and disability insurance, paying monthly cash benefits to more than 64 million people as of 2020 (Social Security Administration 2021a). These various forms of cash payments to Americans have had a significant impact on mental health in the United States.

Many studies have shown a link between economic status and mental health, with general agreement that lower economic status correlates with a higher risk of mental disorders (Hudson 2005; Lund et al. 2010). Although the literature supporting an association between economic status and mental health is substantial, it is difficult to conclusively establish causation, given that practical and ethical limitations on this type of research generally preclude true experiments. The relationship between economic status and mental health is almost certainly, to some degree, bidirectional, a situation often explained by two theories. The *social causation* theory posits that the psychological stress and deprivation associated with lower economic status lead to an increased incidence of mental health disorders (Costello et al. 2003; Golberstein 2015; Sareen et al. 2011). On the other hand, the *social selection* theory posits an inverse relationship, one in which the effects of mental health disorders (e.g., hospitalizations, difficulty maintaining employment) negatively affect an individual's ability to earn money. Furthermore, economic status is closely correlated with other factors related to mental health, such as educational attainment, employment status, access to health care, parental involvement, and neighborhood and community characteristics, making it even more difficult to distinguish the specific effect of economic status on mental health. A decrease in income has been linked to an increased risk of mental disorders, including one finding that adults who experience a reduction in income have increased risk of anxiety, mood, and substance use disorders (Sareen et al. 2011). Moreover, studies have consistently shown an inverse association between economic status and the risk of poor mental health—the lower one's economic status is, the higher one's risk for various mental disorders is (Hudson 2005; Santiago et al. 2011).

For this reason, the widespread insurance-based income programs created by the Social Security Act likely had a population-level protective effect on mental health. These benefits, including Social Security OASDI payments and unemployment insurance, are designed to partially offset reductions in income caused by lost earnings (due to job loss, retirement, death, or disability). One study has even showed that initial unemployment insurance claims may be linked with reduced psychological distress (Tefft 2011).

Studies have specifically examined the effect of Social Security retirement benefits on mental health in older adults, taking advantage of a policy anomaly (the *Social Security notch*) created by amendments to the Social Security Act. Specifically, the 1972 Social Security Amendments created a system of automatic annual cost of living adjustments so that Congress would no longer need to pass individual legislation to account for inflation. However, the formula used in the 1972 amendments was flawed and caused benefits to increase faster than inflation. The statute was amended again in 1977 to correct this error, but Congress chose not to reduce payments for retirees who were already collecting benefits on the basis of the flawed formula. This meant that individuals born prior to 1917 were entitled to significantly higher benefit amounts, even for those with work histories identical to those of individuals born after 1917. This policy anomaly has created the opportunity for quasi-experimental studies. Researchers from the Center for Retirement Research at Boston College, for example, found that the higher benefit levels attributable to the notch were associated with improved cognitive function and improved ability to carry out daily activities (Ayyagari 2015). The same study also found that higher benefits were correlated with a decrease in depressive symptoms within households in which the Social Security recipient had less than a high school education. Another study using data from individuals in the Social Security notch found that the increased retirement income received by those born prior to 1917 significantly improved depressive symptoms and reduced the likelihood of a psychiatric diagnosis for older women (Golberstein 2015).

Social Security's OASDI program lifts between 22 and 27 million Americans out of poverty each year, depending on which measure of poverty is used (Romig 2018). Although OASDI does not specifically target those living in poverty, it has a greater effect on reducing poverty than any other government benefits program. The SSI program helps bring nearly 3 million Americans above the Supplemental Poverty Measure, and TANF and unemployment insurance lift another 400,000 above this floor (Fox 2019). (The Supplemental Poverty Measure is a relatively new standard for measuring poverty and economic conditions that takes into account expenditures for basic necessities and benefits from safety net programs.) Research suggests that the anti-poverty effects of programs arising out of the Social Security Act are likely to lead to improved mental health. Children who grow up consistently poor have worse mental and behavioral health than their better-off peers (Comeau and Boyle 2017), whereas children in families whose income is raised above the poverty level see a reduction in psychiatric symptoms (Costello et al. 2003). Similarly, a family's transition into poverty has been associated with worse mental health for both children and mothers (Wickham et al. 2017). There-fore, if the receipt of any cash benefits through Social Security, SSI, unem-ployment insurance, or TANF prevents a family from entering poverty, it would be protective of the entire family's mental health.

Compared with Social Security's OASDI benefits, other benefits programs arising out of the Social Security Act provide subsistence-level or even lower amounts of financial assistance. Today, benefits through the SSI and TANF programs are available only to those with minimal or no income, and therefore, people in receipt of these benefits by definition have extremely low incomes and are likely to remain below the official poverty level, which, as discussed above, is linked with poor mental health. However, some studies suggest that even among families that remain poor, an increase in income is correlated with a reduction in certain mental health symptoms. Maternal depression among poor, rural families in Mexico was reduced as a result of a decrease in extreme poverty caused by participation in a conditional cash transfer program (Ozer et al. 2011). Similarly, a longitudinal study of a diverse and representative sam-ple of low-income Colorado families found that with respect to symptoms of anxiety and depression, "income levels matter even among a constrained low-income sample," meaning that when it comes to mental health measures, being somewhat poor is still better than being extremely poor (Santiago et al. 2011, p. 227). This is also consistent with a study involving low-income families across the United States that found that in families experiencing "extreme pov-erty" (defined as household income of $9,999 or below per year), caregivers were significantly more likely to experience depression and children were sig-nificantly more likely to exhibit disruptive behavioral disorders than those in families with annual incomes at or above $10,000 (Acri et al. 2017). This sup-ports the idea that although the payment amounts for many of the pro-grams created by the Social Security Act—in particular the means-tested programs such as SSI and TANF—may be too low to actually lift an indi-vidual or family out of poverty, the income from these programs still likely has a positive effect on the mental health of recipients and their families.

Although significant room for improvement remains, the programs that have their roots in the Social Security Act of 1935 did and still do provide a minimal level of income and income stability to many who did not previ-ously have that. By doing so, the Social Security Act has had a significant effect on mental health throughout the country.

Uncertain Future of Social Security Act Programs

As described briefly earlier, the programs with their foundations in the 1935 Social Security Act have undergone a number of significant changes over the past nine decades. Initially, many of the programs were expanded to cover more people or to provide more generous benefits. Over the past few decades, however, concern over the amount of money spent on benefits and entitlements has been a common refrain from many political leaders.

One frequently cited cause for alarm is the impending insolvency of the Social Security trust funds. Although there is some reason for concern about the long-term solvency of the Social Security trust funds, the political rhetoric on this issue has often been overblown and purposefully confusing. The Social Security trust funds support only the federal OASDI programs, with one trust for old-age and survivors insurance and a separate trust for disability insurance. SSI, TANF, unemployment insurance, and other programs and services arising out of the Social Security Act are not funded by the trusts, although they are still frequently the subject of partisan attacks. Because of shifting demographics and the retiring of baby boomers, the OASDI program may eventually be paying out more in benefits each year than the annual tax revenues supporting it. Under current projections, the combined trusts' reserves may be depleted by around 2035; however, even if that occurs, the ongoing annual income from current taxes would be sufficient to cover nearly 79% of benefits payable (Social Security and Medicare Board of Trustees 2020). Considered separately, the most recent estimates show that the old-age and survivor's insurance trust fund can pay full benefits until 2034 and then 76% of benefits payable after that, whereas the disability insurance trust fund can pay full benefits through 2065 (13 years later than the previous report) and then 92% of benefits thereafter (AARP 2021). Moreover, there are legislative proposals that would significantly improve Social Security's financial outlook. President Joseph R. Biden's plan to strengthen Social Security with a modest expansion of the Social Security tax base not only would extend the Social Security trust fund reserves but also would allow for a variety of increases in benefit amounts (Favreault 2020).

The idea of "privatizing" Social Security has been discussed for decades, perhaps most intensely during the presidency of George W. Bush. The basic idea behind privatization is to replace part or all of the current publicly administered and tax-funded Social Security program with individual retirement savings accounts that would be invested and individually managed. Proponents of privatization argue that it would allow for higher returns on the accounts as invested, resulting in higher payouts for retired workers compared with Social Security. However, privatization could require significant compromises with respect to workers who are currently receiving benefits or nearing retirement age, and because the accounts would be invested, they would be subject to the volatility of the stock market. In addition, the obligation to manage an individual retirement account, including making decisions about investment strategies, would be particularly burdensome or impossible for many Social Security beneficiaries, especially those of older age or with certain mental disorders. Improper management of an account would threaten the financial security of those already predisposed to less economic stability. Although many Republican politicians supported privatization, the proposal failed to gain significant public support and ultimately failed to pass, despite it being a key policy goal during both of George W. Bush's terms.

Recognizing that Social Security remains a popular program among most Americans, Donald J. Trump promised to protect Social Security during his presidential campaign. Despite these promises, many Republicans still hoped to make cuts to Social Security, including reductions in benefits (Tankersley and Cochrane 2019). In his 2020 budget proposal, President Trump himself proposed cutting approximately $25 billion from Social Security's annual budget, including significant cuts to disability benefits, significant reductions in SSI benefits payable for many individuals, and reductions in funding for Social Security's administrative costs (National Committee to Preserve Social Security and Medicare 2019). Although Trump failed to win reelection, such continued proposals demonstrate Social Security's continued vulnerability. Any proposal that would decrease cash benefit amounts would increase poverty rates and could have potentially harmful consequences on the mental health of current and future recipients. On the basis of their study of the effects of the Social Security notch and the difference in benefit calculations, researchers at Boston College specifically concluded that "cuts to Social Security benefits could potentially have significant negative impacts on the functional limitations and cognitive function of older adults, while increases in benefits could lead to improvements in health outcomes" (Ayyagari 2015).

Social Security benefits themselves are not the only programs created by the Social Security Act that have been placed under threat. Proposed "entitlement reform" has taken aim at a number of other programs as well. Many proposals have sought to impose more and stricter requirements for means-tested programs that tend to assist those with lower incomes. TANF and Medicaid are common targets. Such changes would certainly have a negative population-level impact on mental health. Adding or expanding work requirements is a common element of reform proposals, yet imposing additional work requirements to receive benefits in the past has had the effect of significantly reducing the number of people who receive these subsistence benefits without a similar increase in employment for those who were or would previously have been eligible for assistance (Pavetti 2018). People with mental health conditions, who are more likely to rely on benefit programs, often have difficulty complying with work requirements, putting them at greater risk of having their assistance reduced or terminated (Danziger et al. 2009). On the basis of the research discussed above (Hudson 2005; Santiago et al. 2011; Sareen et al. 2011), this loss of income could contribute to worse mental health and/or exacerbations of mental illnesses for those affected.

The Social Security Act of 1935 laid the foundation for what would become the country's most important safety net programs. Arising from the desperation of the Great Depression and resulting from the enduring commitment of Frances Perkins and other patriots like her, the act became embedded into our national consciousness: a conviction that when great numbers of Americans find themselves in need, the federal government has a role to play in their financial aid and security. And in soothing economic anxieties, it has played and will doubtless continue to play a key role in supporting mental wellness and preventing mental illnesses in the U.S. population. We owe it to both the legacy of those who fought for the Social Security Act and its subsequent improvements, as well as future generations of Americans, to protect it and even advocate for enhanced benefits.

References

AARP: Social Security combined trust funds projection remains the same says board of trustees. Washington, DC, AARP, 2021. Available at: https://states.aarp.org/virginia/social-security-combined-trust-funds-projection-remains-the-same-says-board-of-trustees. Accessed May 11, 2021.

Acri MC, Bornheimer LA, Jessell L, et al: The intersection of extreme poverty and familial mental health in the United States. Soc Work Ment Health 15(6):677–689, 2017 29618956

Aid to homeless over nation set a new high in February. The New York Times, May 15, 1933. Available at: https://timesmachine.nytimes.com/timesmachine/1933/05/15/105136157.pdf. Accessed May 11, 2021.

An Act to Amend Title IV of the Social Security Act to Authorize Federal Financial Participation in Aid to Dependent Children of Unemployed Parents, and for Other Purposes of 1961, Pub. L. No. 87-31.

Ayyagari P: Evaluating the impact of social security benefits on health outcomes among the elderly. Boston, Center for Retirement Research, Boston College, September 2015. Available at: https://collections.nlm.nih.gov/master/borndig/101705940/wp_2015-25.pdf. Accessed May 11, 2021.

Becker A: Factbox: what Republicans mean when they talk about U.S. welfare reform. Reuters, January 8, 2018. Available at: www.reuters.com/article/us-usa-congress-welfare-factbox/factbox-what-republicans-mean-when-they-talk-about-u-s-welfare-reform-idUSKBN1EX1ZZ. Accessed May 11, 2021.

Comeau J, Boyle MH: Patterns of poverty exposure and children's trajectories of externalizing and internalizing behaviors. SSM Popul Health 4:86–94, 2017 29349277

Costello EJ, Compton SN, Keeler G, et al: Relationships between poverty and psychopathology: a natural experiment. JAMA 290(15):2023–2029, 2003 14559956

Danziger S, Frank RG, Meara E: Mental illness, work, and income support programs. Am J Psychiatry 166(4):398–404, 2009 19339364

Disputes Hoover on employment. The New York Times, January 23, 1930. Available at: https://timesmachine.nytimes.com/timesmachine/1930/01/23/94233187.pdf. Accessed May 11, 2021.

Doctor's plan of guaranteed aid started it. Los Angeles Times, August 12, 1985. Available at: www.latimes.com/archives/la-xpm-1985-08-12-mn-3999-story.html. Accessed May 11, 2021.

Downey K: The Woman Behind the New Deal: The Life of Frances Perkins, FDR's Secretary of Labor and His Moral Conscience. New York, Anchor, 2009

Ellis N: Survivors of the Great Depression tell their stories. Washington, DC, NPR, November 27, 2008. Available at: www.npr.org/templates/story/story.php?storyId=97468008. Accessed May 11, 2021.

Favreault M: A close look at Joe Biden's Social Security proposals. Washington, DC, Tax Policy Center, 2020. Available at: www.taxpolicycenter.org/taxvox/close-look-joe-bidens-social-security-proposals. Accessed May 11, 2021.

Foote RO: Pensions for all at 60: an idea from the West. The New York Times, September 16, 1934. Available at: https://timesmachine.nytimes.com/timesmachine/1934/09/16/93767525.pdf. Accessed May 11, 2021.

Fox L: The supplemental poverty measure: 2018. Suitland, MD, U.S. Census Bureau, October 7, 2019. Available at: www.census.gov/library/publications/2019/demo/p60-268.html. Accessed February 7, 2022.

Golberstein E: The effects of income on mental health: evidence from the social security notch. J Ment Health Policy Econ 18(1):27–37, 2015 25862202

Hiltzik M: The New Deal: A Modern History. New York, Simon & Schuster, 2011

Hudson CG: Socioeconomic status and mental illness: tests of the social causation and selection hypotheses. Am J Orthopsychiatry 75(1):3–18, 2005 15709846

Lund C, Breen A, Flisher AJ, et al: Poverty and common mental disorders in low and middle income countries: a systematic review. Soc Sci Med 71(3):517–528, 2010 20621748

McElvaine RS: The Depression and New Deal: A History in Documents. New York, Oxford University Press, 2000

National Committee to Preserve Social Security and Medicare: The president's FY 2020 budget: it literally leaves seniors in the cold. Washington, DC, National Committee to Preserve Social Security and Medicare, March 22, 2019. Available at: www.ncpssm.org/documents/medicaid-policy-papers/the-presidents-fy-2020-budget-it-literally-leaves-seniors-in-the-cold. Accessed May 11, 2021.

New York Codes, Rules, and Regulations, Title 18, Section 352 (2020)

1,250,000 homeless reported in nation. The New York Times, February 17, 1933. Available at: https://timesmachine.nytimes.com/timesmachine/1933/02/17/99293619.pdf. Accessed May 11, 2021.

Ozer EJ, Fernald LC, Weber A, et al: Does alleviating poverty affect mothers' depressive symptoms? A quasi-experimental investigation of Mexico's Oportunidades programme. Int J Epidemiol 40(6):1565–1576, 2011 21737404

Pavetti L: TANF studies show work requirement proposals for other programs would harm millions, do little to increase work. Washington, DC, Center on Budget and Policy Priorities, November 13, 2018. Available at: www.cbpp.org/sites/default/files/atoms/files/11-13-18tanf.pdf. Accessed May 11, 2021.

Pension proposal called fantastic. The New York Times, November 7, 1934. Available at: https://timesmachine.nytimes.com/timesmachine/1934/11/07/94579620.pdf. Accessed May 11, 2021.

Perkins F: The roots of Social Security. Remarks presented at the Social Security Administration headquarters, Baltimore, MD, October 23, 1962. Available at: https://awpc.cattcenter.iastate.edu/2017/03/21/the-roots-of-social-security-oct-23-1962. Accessed May 11, 2021.

Personal Responsibility and Work Opportunity Reconciliation Act of 1996, Pub. L. 104–193.

Piven FF, Cloward R: Regulating the Poor: The Functions of Public Welfare. New York, Vintage, 2012

President's Committee on Economic Security: The Program for Economic Security. Washington, DC, President's Committee on Economic Security, 1935. Available at: www.ssa.gov/history/reports/ces/cesvol9program.html. Accessed May 11, 2021.

Public Welfare Amendments of 1962. Pub. L. 87–543.

Rodems R, Shaefer H: Left out: policy diffusion and the exclusion of Black workers from unemployment insurance. Soc Sci Hist 40(3):385–404, 2016

Romig K: Social Security lifts more Americans above poverty than any other program. Washington, DC, Center on Budget and Policy Priorities, 2018. Available at: www.cbpp.org/sites/default/files/atoms/files/10-25-13ss.pdf. Accessed May 11, 2021.

Santiago CD, Wadsworth M, Stump J: Socioeconomic status, neighborhood disadvantage, and poverty-related stress: prospective effects on psychological syndromes among diverse low-income families. J Econ Psychol 32(2):218–230, 2011

Sareen J, Afifi TO, McMillan KA, et al: Relationship between household income and mental disorders: findings from a population-based longitudinal study. Arch Gen Psychiatry 68(4):419–427, 2011 21464366

The security bill. The New York Times, April 21, 1935. Available at: https://timesmachine.nytimes.com/timesmachine/1935/04/21/94601012.pdf. Accessed May 11, 2021.

Security bill challenged. The New York Times, May 4, 1935. Available at: https://timesmachine.nytimes.com/timesmachine/1935/05/04/95502591.pdf. Accessed May 11, 2021.

Social Security Act of 1935, Pub. L. 74-271.

Social Security Act Amendments of 1939, Pub. L. 76-379.

Social Security Act Amendments of 1950, Pub. L. 81-734.

Social Security Administration: SSI annual statistical report 2017. Washington DC, Social Security Administration, July 2018. Available at: www.ssa.gov/policy/docs/statcomps/ssi_asr/2017/index.html. Accessed February 7, 2022.

Social Security Administration: Social security beneficiary statistics. Washington DC, Social Security Administration, 2021a. Available at: www.ssa.gov/oact/STATS/OASDIbenies.html. Accessed May 11, 2021.

Social Security Administration: SSI federal payment amounts for 2021. Washington DC, Social Security Administration, 2021b. Available at: www.ssa.gov/oact/cola/SSI.html. Accessed May 11, 2021.

Social Security Amendments of 1954, Pub. L. 83-761.

Social Security Amendments of 1956, Pub. L. 84-880.

Social Security Amendments of 1967, Pub. L. 90-248.

Social Security Amendments of 1972, Pub. L. 92-603.

Social Security Amendments of 1983, Pub. L. 98-21.

Social Security and Medicare Board of Trustees: Status of the Social Security and Medicare programs. Washington DC, Social Security Administration, 2020. Available at: www.ssa.gov/oact/TRSUM/#:~:text=In%202019%2C%20Social%20Security's%20reserves,2034%2C%20unchanged%20from%20last%20year. Accessed May 11, 2021.

Sprague LW: Her life: the woman behind the New Deal. Newcastle, ME, Frances Perkins Center, June 1, 2014. Available at: http://francesperkinscenter.org/life-new. Accessed May 11, 2021.

Stark L: Hopes are fading for security bill. The New York Times, March 20, 1935a. Available at: www.nytimes.com/2019/08/21/us/politics/deficit-will-reach-1-trillion-next-year-budget-office-predicts.html?smid=nytcore-ios-share. Accessed May 11, 2021.

Stark L: Wagner Social Security plan attacked by experts as "hazy." The New York Times, January 20, 1935b. Available at: http://timesmachine.nytimes.com/timesmachine/1935/01/20/93443276.pdf. Accessed May 11, 2021.

Tankersley J, Cochrane E: Budget deficit on path to surpass $1 trillion under Trump. The New York Times, August 21, 2019. Available at: www.nytimes.com/2019/08/21/us/politics/deficit-will-reach-1-trillion-next-year-budget-office-predicts.html?smid=nytcore-ios-share. Accessed May 11, 2021.

Tefft N: Insights on unemployment, unemployment insurance, and mental health. J Health Econ 30(2):258–264, 2011 21349596

Wickham S, Whitehead M, Taylor-Robinson D, et al: The effect of a transition into poverty on child and maternal mental health: a longitudinal analysis of the UK Millennium Cohort Study. Lancet Public Health 2(3):e141–e148, 2017 29253387

5 | Clearing the Air for Mental Health

The Clean Air Act of 1963

Benson S. Ku, M.D.
Elizabeth Haase, M.D.

A Rude Awakening

On Wednesday, October 27, 1948, several thousand people in Donora, Pennsylvania, were injured, and dozens died suffering. The acrid, yellowish-gray blanket that smothered the mill town in southwestern Pennsylvania, just south of Pittsburgh, was more suffocating than anything any Donoran had ever seen—or inhaled. "It was so bad," Jerry Campa, a Donoran restaurateur recalled, "that I'd accidentally step off the curb and turn my ankle because I couldn't see my feet" (Kiester 1999). The smog was so intense that Dr. William Rongaus, the head of the local board of health, suggested that all residents with preexisting respiratory problems immediately leave town (History.com 2009; https://sphweb.bumc.bu.edu/otlt/MPH-Modules/PH/RespiratoryHealth/Temperature%20Inversion%20iFrame.html).

However, residents who attempted to evacuate mostly failed, primarily because of the visibility impairment that the heavy smog caused. In fact, driving was nearly abandoned. "I drove on the left side of the street with my head out the window...steering by scraping the curb," recalled Russell Davis, who was working at the Donora Fire Department (Kiester 1999).

The people of Donora were also struggling to *breathe*. "About 4 o'clock Friday," Eileen Loftus, a nurse at the American Steel and Wire Company, recalled, "a worker staggered in, gasping. I had him lie down and gave him oxygen. Then another man came in, and another" (Kiester 1999). By early evening, every bed and examining table in the two local hospitals were occupied by a wheezing and often panicky worker. So many people required help that an emergency hospital was temporarily set up in a hotel. The first death occurred that same day.

By Saturday, the three funeral homes had more corpses than they could handle. The town had set up a temporary morgue underneath the emergency hospital because the funeral directors were overwhelmed by the number of bodies. The eight doctors in the town, who belonged to the Donora Medical Association, made house calls much like the firefighters in town, visiting anyone who called for help. People were calling every doctor they could with the hope of getting treatment faster. It was not until midday Saturday that Cora Vernon, executive director of Donora's Red Cross, redirected all calls going to the doctors' offices to the emergency center.

Before a rainstorm washed the noxious smog away a few days later, 20 people had died, and nearly half the population was sickened. Another 50 residents died of respiratory illness within a month after the incident. Notable among the fatalities was Lukasz Musial, the father of future baseball Hall of Famer Stan Musial, the 1948 National League's most valuable player (Holmes 2012). The environmental disaster in Donora shocked the entire nation and forever changed the way Americans thought about industrial pollution and health.

Donora, a town of 14,000 people, was home to steel mills and a zinc smelting plant that had released excessive amounts of sulfuric acid, carbon monoxide, and other pollutants into the atmosphere for years prior to the disaster (Figure 5–1). During the 1920s, the owner of the zinc plant, Zinc Works, compensated local residents for damages caused by the pollution. However, not everyone was quick to blame the steel mills and zinc plants as the culprit of the disaster. In fact, Marcia Spink, former associate director for air programs for the U.S. Environmental Protection Agency's (EPA) Region III office in Philadelphia, remembered that before this incident, "people thought of smog as a nuisance. It made your shirts dirty.... When I was growing up in western Pennsylvania, grime and dirty air were facts of life. We walked home for lunch with streetlights still blazing; my mother washed the living-room curtains almost every week" (Kiester 1999). Residents were used to pollution from the town's cluster of industries that formed the bedrock of the region's economy—making steel, wire, and nails. Charles Stacey, a long-time resident, teacher, and local historian, offered similar opinions regarding Donorans' attitudes on smog. He told *In These*

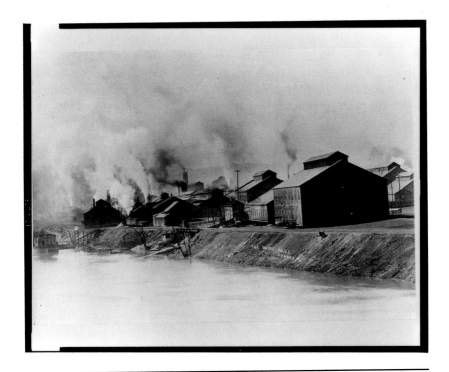

FIGURE 5–1.   **Wire mills spewing smoke along the Monongahela River, Donora, Pennsylvania.**
Source.   Dresbach B: "The wire mill, Donora, PA," 1910. Library of Congress, Prints & Photographs Division, LC-USZ62-131258. Copyright by Bruce Dresbach, Donora, PA. Available at: www.loc.gov/resource/cph.3c31258. Accessed February 8, 2022.

Times, a nonprofit magazine, "They were used to plumes of smoke billowing into the sky and seeing everything covered in red dust from the iron ore used to make steel" (Lydersen 2014).

At that time, "memories of the Great Depression were still vivid, and smog meant prosperity," Spink added (Kiester 1999). Although the smog became the subject of national outrage and media attention, steel and zinc mills employed about 5,000 of the town's 14,000 inhabitants, and Stacey noted that many people in Donora were reluctant to point fingers. Stacey observed, "They thought if the mills were blamed, they would shut down, and Donora would lose its prosperity. People wanted to put this behind them and go back to their jobs" (Lydersen 2014). As a result, there was little, if any, regulation of the air pollution caused by the industries of Donora. Even after the incident of October 27, the steel mill and the zinc plants continued to operate, stacks steadily spewing more fumes into the heavily polluted atmosphere. The zinc mills finally halted operations 4 days later, following several days of public pleas to shut down. Rain fell soon afterward, and the air began to clear. Even after temporarily stopping operations for "precautionary measures," officials at U.S. Steel Corp., owner of the mills, maintained that the situation was unlikely to be caused by their operations, declaring that the zinc mills had been safely using the same procedures since 1915.

Over the next several months, state and federal investigators interviewed every third household. They also set up air quality monitoring sites, checked medical records and vital statistics, and brought in meteorological and biological research teams. In 1949, the U.S. Public Health Service issued a 173-page report, "Air Pollution in Donora, Pa.: Epidemiology of the Unusual Smog Episode of October 1948" (Schrenk and Mountin 1949). Although the report counted 5,910 people affected by the smog, it failed to identify a definite culprit. Donora's topography and abnormal weather pattern were primarily blamed. Not surprisingly, the report was highly criticized. Critics noted that the permissible emission levels were for healthy young workers in the plants, not older or medically ill people in the community. Those who passed away from the smog had all been age 52 or older, most with heart or lung problems. Vindicating the zinc mills outraged many people. A local newspaper declared, "You didn't need science to identify the culprit, just a pair of reasonably good eyes" (ExplorePAhistory.com 2019). Around 100 lawsuits—later settled in 1951 for a total of $256,000 without assessing blame—were filed against American Steel and Wire. Citizens' groups started to demand stiffer smog regulation.

Investigations would later confirm that a temperature inversion, a layer of warm air hovering above the valley, had prevented the dissipation of air pollution from the mills on that particular day—specifically the pollution from Donora Zinc Works, which produced a toxic blend of sulfuric acid, nitrogen dioxide, fluoride, and other compounds (Ivel 2017). Despite pressure from steel and mill companies to withdraw research publications that showed harmful effects of smog, extensive research showed that pollutants from the zinc plant contributed to injury and death. Fluorine gas generated in the zinc smelting process was trapped by the stagnant air and was the primary cause of the deaths. Dr. Devra L. Davis, director of the Center for Environmental Oncology at the University of Pittsburgh Cancer Institute, showed that fluorine levels in victims were in the lethal range, as much as 20 times higher than normal in autopsy results (Hopey 2008).

The smog was a wake-up call about the dangers of industrial air pollution. Quickly following this terrifying event, investigations and research led to effective changes. In 1950, President Harry S. Truman convened the first national air pollution conference, citing Donora as an example of the need.

Donora's mills and zinc works ultimately closed in the 1950s and 1960s, soon followed by the decline of the U.S. steel industry that swept the nation. Thirteen years later, in 1963, the first Clean Air Act (CAA) was signed, establishing a legal obligation to protect Americans from pollutants that endanger their health or welfare. The signing of the CAA and subsequent amendments was driven not only by the disastrous impacts of air pollution, including the Donora smog, but also by U.S. citizens and political figures working together to voice their concerns about the detrimental health impacts of air pollution and fiercely advocating for cleaner air. The passage of the CAA represents the powerful impact that visible air pollution had on moving political will.

Edmund Muskie: A Visionary Leader

The Donora smog, along with other tragic incidents causing pollution-related deaths in London and New York, led to the passage of the Air Pollution Control Act of 1955. Although this act did little to set targets for air pollution, it served as the platform for Congress to pass the first federal standard for air quality, championed by Senator Edmund S. Muskie—who would later be secretary of state—(Figure 5–2), who has been heralded as the "father of the modern environmental movement" (Billings 2000) and "our most important environmental leader" (Billings 1996). His legacy endures in environmental laws such as the CAA and Clean Water Act, pieces of environmental legislation that have protected public health and life for more than 50 years. These laws have had a stunningly positive impact on the nation's natural environment. It takes little imagination to speculate what our national landscape would now look like if the economic growth over the past five decades had not been accompanied by the environmental protections the laws provided.

Edmund Muskie grew up in Rumford, Maine, and from an early age, he observed the effects that pollution from nearby paper mill smokestacks had on the local air and the Androscoggin River. In his 1954 gubernatorial campaign, his environmental platform argued for the creation of antipollution legislation. As governor, he called for legislation to address water pollution and began to confront the complexity of the problem. In April 1963, Muskie became the chairman of the newly created Senate Subcommittee on Air and Water Pollution. Muskie quickly commissioned comprehensive staff reports on water and air pollution. Early on, Muskie saw that pollution was interfering with economic development as well as public health. By mid-June 1963, Muskie was holding 6 days of hearings on water pollution and 3 days of hearings on air pollution, which culminated in the Senate passing legislation in both areas that year (Goldstein 2015).

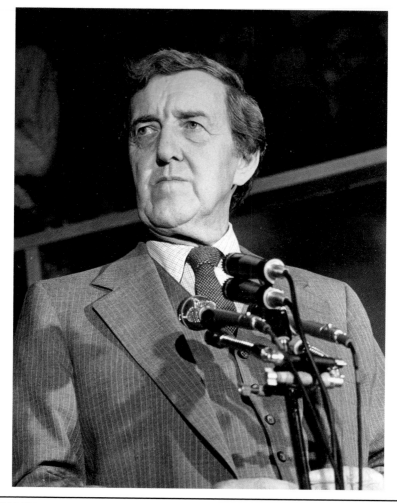

FIGURE 5–2.   **Secretary of State Edmund Muskie.**
This photograph was taken during a State Department farewell event at the end of the Carter administration.
Source.   U.S. National Archives: "Secretary of State Edmund Muskie, Who Presided over the Latest U.S. Government Internal Debate over Reprocessing Policy During the Summer of 1980." U.S. National Archives, Still Pictures Unit, RG 59-SE, Box 8. Available at: https://nsarchive.gwu.edu/sites/default/files/thumbnails/image/photo-3-3.jpg. Accessed May 13, 2022.

The work of this great American environmental legislation leader required mastery of every aspect of the subject—technical, political, strategic, and constitutional. From his first term in the Senate onward, Muskie was deeply immersed in issues related to federalism and intergovernmental matters, and by the mid-1960s, if not before, he was widely recognized by close congressional observers as one of the Senate's most capable and constructive members. Later, after Vietnam and Watergate, Muskie became involved in issues related to the separation of powers. As the first chair of the Senate Budget Committee, Muskie led Congress to exercise its spending power in a more coherent fashion as he managed the War Powers Resolution and became intricately involved in foreign policy.

Muskie's strong commitment to serving the public interest included protecting the health and welfare of individuals. He rejected arguments that economic growth and protecting the environment were necessarily at odds with each other. "An economic growth policy which abandons environmental objectives would be a foolish course. The nation must have clean growth," he announced to the Senate in 1976 (Goldstein 2015, p. 230). Muskie recognized that pollution contributed substantial costs, and he did not believe that economic gain justified polluting the earth or poisoning people. Leon Billings noted that Muskie studied environmental issues intensely and extensively. At times, Muskie had to operate with little scientific information, but when data were available, he collected, studied, internalized, and acted on them (Billings 2015; Goldstein 2015).

An extraordinary quality of Muskie was his ability to collaborate. As a legislator, he has been compared with a symphony conductor rather than a soloist (Goldstein 2015). Muskie collected and included the best suggestions of his colleagues. Thus, the CAA reflected Senator Howard Baker's (R-TN) belief that technology could be harnessed to reduce air pollution, Senator Tom Eagleton's (D-MO) commitment to deadlines as a necessary ingredient of laws that would deliver on promises, and Muskie's insistence that environmental law safeguard human health. Muskie knew both when to walk away from negotiations to force concessions and how to compromise effectively to fuel legislative accomplishment. Although committed to the purity of his environmental positions, he knew when to enact partial advances rather than lose. He was aware that legislation was a collaborative process and, accordingly, that accommodation and consensus were its necessary ingredients.

As collaborative as he was, Muskie was not without opposition. The National Air Quality Standards Act of 1970, an amendment to the CAA of 1963 composed by Senator Muskie and his subcommittee, required that by 1975 (later postponed to 1978), automobiles achieve a 90% reduction of the 1970 standards for emissions of carbon monoxide, hydrocarbons, and nitrogen oxides. Although this amendment had wide support, it was criticized for lack of technological feasibility and high costs. Senator Robert P. Griffin (R-MI), along with members of the auto industry, including Edward N. Cole, president of the General Motors Corporation, spoke at length against the bill. Their opposition maintained that it was not technologically feasible to meet the 1975 deadline and that "cleaning up auto emissions would raise the price of cars" (Kenworthy 1970, p. 24). However, the EPA successfully forced the adoption of two marquee control technologies: the catalytic converter in 1975 and the three-way catalyst in 1981 (Gerard and Lave 2005), novel technologies that reduced air pollutant emissions and helped the companies achieve the targeted standards. In response to criticism about the cost of reducing auto emissions, Muskie replied, "Where would the Senator place a decision of such importance to the public health? In the boards of directors of 'these great motor companies?' Does Congress have no responsibility?" (Congressional Record 1970). A retrospective analysis of the benefits and costs of implementing the CAA from 1970 to 1990 indicates that the mean estimate of total benefits over the period exceeded total costs by more than a factor of 42 (U.S. Environmental Protection Agency 2017a).

The enduring nature of Edmund Muskie's legislation testifies to his commitment, integrity, and passion for improving the environment. Decades after enactment of the CAA, the basic legal architecture of this act and its amendments remains largely intact. Although some members of Congress have repeatedly attempted to dismantle that architecture, they have mostly failed. And although Congress in recent decades has distanced itself from environmental lawmaking and Muskie himself has departed from those legislative chambers, his voice is still present in the CAA, which has withstood several Supreme Court challenges and is the backbone of efforts to combat the climate change threats facing the world today. His voice, expressed in the arguments made by lawyers and in the judicial rulings themselves—especially in the EPA's current efforts to invoke its CAA authorities to address the worldwide threat of climate change—had withstood several challenges in court, including the Supreme Court, but whether this voice will continue to stand the test of time has recently come into serious question.

On the Road to Cleaner Air

The CAA, the details of which will be described in the next section, has had strong impacts on virtually all facets of human life in the United States, from industries such as automobile manufacturing and sales to human health and preservation of the environment. However, these powerful effects did not occur overnight but stemmed from the evolution of the act itself, following a long process involving many environmental disasters, political proponents and detractors, and vocal advocacy groups. Although public health officials expressed concerns about the detrimental health effects of air pollution as early as the 1940s, it was not until two other major environmental disasters occurred following the Donora smog event—the Great Smog of

London in December 1952, in which sulfurous smog killed about 4,000 people in 1 week, and a similar incident in New York City in 1953 that resulted in 200 deaths—that outrage over tragic pollution-related fatalities prompted passage of the 1955 Air Pollution Control Act. Following World War II, the 1955 act also represented a shift of American values from national and economic security toward quality-of-life issues, including the health of the environment.

In March 1963, the House Health and Safety Subcommittee heard 2 days of testimony on whether the federal government should expand its air pollution program to include new enforcement authorities proposed in the CAA. For the first time, opponents of the federal air pollution legislation presented their arguments in this forum. Opposition came from the government and industries (Orford 2021). From the government, states were wary that municipal-federal dealings would undercut the states' powers. They argued that the bill should focus solely on promoting interstate cooperation, rather than providing "machinery for ousting of local and State jurisdiction...on the basis of administrative discretion" (Orford 2021, p. 151). Industries were particularly hostile to the CAA and emphasized that "cooperative community action" alone was sufficient to combat air pollution effectively. Moreover, the National Association of Manufacturers argued that the new water pollution control paradigm had problems and should not be expanded too hastily to the air pollution control context.

Following the hearing, the CAA's sponsors in the House of Representatives revised the bill, making minor amendments, including several additional checks on the federal government's enforcement authority in response to hearing comments, but was almost entirely unresponsive to the statements of the states' and industries' opposition. The bill passed the House after a vigorous debate and was then sent to the Senate, where it arrived before Senator Muskie's newly formed Special Subcommittee on Air and Water Pollution. Muskie fiercely confronted the industry representatives on the positions discussed above, an aggressive tactic that took them by surprise (Orford 2021).

After the House and Senate passed the CAA, President Lyndon B. Johnson signed it into law on December 17, 1963. This act, which was the first act to authorize federal government regulation over major sources of pollution, helped establish a powerful model of policy-making as a continuous, dynamic process of identifying problems, formulating government responses, organizing administrative mechanisms for carrying out the policies, and evaluating the effectiveness of the government response.

The CAA and its amendments evolved from a complex historical interplay of environmental disasters, public support, advocacy from environmentalists, and collaboration among politicians. Although this evolution has already resulted in dramatic improvement in air quality and public health, the shift in attention to global climate change now calls for further legislative action.

Clean Air Act of 1963

The CAA, which Congress passed on December 17, 1963, was the first major piece of federal legislation on air pollution control. The act began with identifying various sources of air pollution, including "urbanization, industrial development, and...motor vehicles" (Clean Air Act of 1963). It then set forth specific and detailed purposes to "(1) protect the Nation's air resources..., (2) initiate and accelerate a national research and development program..., (3) provide technical and financial assistance to State and local governments in connection with...air pollution prevention and control programs, and (4) encourage...regional air pollution control programs." In Section 2, the act encouraged cooperative activities not only between state and local governments but also among states and federal agencies.

Section 3 required the secretary of health, education, and welfare to establish a national research and development program for the prevention and control of air pollution. This program would conduct general research, provide financial assistance to air pollution control agencies, and set a specific research goal of extracting sulfur from fuels. This section then mandated the secretary to publish "criteria" for informational purposes and make them available to interested parties under certain conditions. That is, if the secretary determined that either a particular agent or combination of air pollution agents was present in the air in certain quantities producing harmful health effects, then the secretary would be required to compile and publish criteria. The criteria were defined as the most up-to-date scientific knowledge of the "kind and extent of [harmful] effects...expected from the presence of such air pollution agent (or combination of agents) in the air in varying quantities." By defining the criteria as entities that would be continuously updated and reflecting the latest scientific knowledge, the emphasis was on identifying criteria and a process to develop air quality standards as new conditions arose, rather than the air quality standards themselves.

The fourth section of the 1963 CAA expanded funding to state and local governments by granting up to two-thirds of the cost of developing, establishing, and improving programs for the prevention and control of air pollution to air pollution control agencies and up to three-quarters of the cost to regional air pollution programs. By offering a higher financial incentive for regional programs, Congress encouraged cooperative approaches among states to resolve issues related to interstate air pollution.

In Section 5, Congress recognized air pollution as an endangerment to the "health, or welfare of any persons." It further specified the Department of Health, Education, and Welfare's authority on the basis of whether air pollution was interstate (air pollution generated in one state that crosses state borders, affecting air quality in another state) or intrastate (polluted air that stays within a state's boundaries), allowing greater exercise of federal authority in the former case compared with the latter. If a state or local government was concerned about a source of interstate air pollution, the secretary would be required to intervene and issue a notice of conference among the interested agencies. To trigger this requirement, the discharge only had to be "causing or contributing to such pollution." The secretary also had authority to call a conference even without a request by a state or local government authority if the secretary believed that air pollution was occurring and was endangering the health and welfare of persons in other states.

In contrast, for concerns regarding intrastate air pollution, the secretary was required to issue a notice of conference only if there was "air pollution which is endangering the health or welfare of persons," a higher standard that requires actual endangerment, not just alleged endangerment. The secretary had the discretion to determine the extent and impact of air pollution impact and whether the pollution was significant enough to warrant exercise of the federal jurisdiction. Along with discretionary duties that allowed the secretary to avoid mandatory obligation to issue a notice of conference, these requirements made it more difficult for the federal government to intervene in the case of intrastate pollution control compared with interstate air pollution. Although it was concerned with the problem of air pollution, Congress was cautious not to infringe on the authority of state and local governments.

The secretary was also granted powers to resolve disputes over interstate and intrastate air pollution. Following a conference procedure, the act specified the course of action and the timeline if the secretary believed there was a lack of effective progress or if there was endangerment to the health and welfare of any persons. This administrative procedure was supported with a judicial enforcement procedure, which laid the foundation for the use of injunctions against interstate pollution in the modern CAA. For intrastate pollution, the secretary was required to provide "technical and other assistance" to a state in judicial proceedings, but federal authority somewhat depended on a state first making a request for assistance.

Section 6 concerned Congress's first significant creation of a federal role to address air pollution from mobile sources, including cars and trucks. It encouraged "the continued efforts [of the] automotive and fuel industry to develop devices and fuels to prevent pollutants from being discharged from the exhaust of automotive vehicles." A technical committee of representatives of automotive vehicle, exhaust control device, and fuel manufacturers was required to meet periodically and "evaluate progress in the development of such devices and fuels and to develop and recommend research programs." The secretary was then required to report to Congress "on measures taken toward the resolution of the vehicle exhaust pollution problem and efforts to improve fuels." Thus, Congress set the framework for an approach to air emissions from mobile sources that contemplated addressing air pollution on the front end through the fuel manufacturer, on the back end through the emissions control device manufacturer, and in the design of the actual vehicle through the automobile manufacturer, allowing regulations of all parts of the fuel-burning cycle.

In Section 7, Congress expressed the intent for federal agencies to have jurisdiction over "building, installation, or other property" and to cooperate with the secretary and with "any air pollution control agency in preventing and controlling the pollution of the air." The terms used in this section would later develop into the single term *stationary source* in the modern CAA, which was defined as "any building structure, facility, or installation." This section also authorized the secretary to identify particular facilities that would be subject to federal air permit requirements, which would later lead to the development of the New Source Performance Standards in 1970. These standards would limit the amount of dangerous emissions American companies could produce.

Section 8 allowed Congress to establish a long-term federal regulatory program for air pollution by authorizing the secretary to "prescribe such regulations as are necessary to carry out his functions under this Act." The next section expanded the definitions of several terms subject to regulation, including "adverse effects on welfare" from the 1955 act. In Section 9, this term's definition expanded to include "injury to agricultural crops and livestock, damage to and the deterioration of property, and hazards to transportation."

Amendments to the Clean Air Act

The 1955 act represented a significant first step in the federal regulation of air pollution, despite its limited focus. Although there were no federal air pollution targets, the 1955 act initiated the authorization of funding for federal-level air pollution research. In addition, the phrase "dangers to the public health and welfare" introduced a new perspective on air pollution that included effects on the public in addition to the individual (Air Pollution Control Act of 1955). Later, *dangers* would evolve into the concept of *endangerment*, which would subsequently function as a condition for triggering mandatory action by the EPA to address a particular air pollutant (Clean

Air Amendments of 1970). The wording "endangerment of public health and welfare" has important implications for policy on health, including mental health. This part of the law is being used in current court cases to justify the regulation of greenhouse gases in order to control the public health impacts of climate change.

In 1969, two oil spills off the California coast and the explosion of flames on the Cuyahoga River in Cleveland captured the attention of the public and contributed to the establishment of the first Earth Day on April 22, 1970. The Earth Day movement brought together 20 million Americans for peaceful demonstrations in favor of environmental policy reform. Air pollution and environmental awareness, heated topics that were highly publicized, increased political will for comprehensive national air quality legislation. In 1970, 70% of Americans agreed that air and water pollution were serious problems where they lived, a huge increase compared with about a third of Americans expressing the same view in 1965 (Rinde 2017). In his State of the Union address to Congress, President Richard Nixon declared, "The great question of the seventies is, shall we surrender to our surroundings, or shall we make peace with nature and begin to make reparations for the damage we have done to our air, to our land, and to our water?" Driven by his rivalry with Senator Muskie in the 1972 presidential election, Nixon called for "comprehensive new regulations" to protect the environment (Augustine 2005; "Transcript of the President's State of the Union" 1970) and signed the Clean Air Amendments of 1970. These amendments were enacted by Congress 4 weeks after the National Environmental Policy Act established the EPA and resulted in a major expansion in the federal government's role in air pollution control.

It was fortuitous that these amendments were enacted at that political moment because after Nixon was elected, it became clear that he was apathetic about the environment and had supported environmental policies only for political reasons. In 1972, Nixon vetoed the Clean Water Act, stating that the act was just too expensive. Muskie responded, "Can we afford clean water? Can we afford rivers and lakes and streams and oceans which continue to make life possible on this planet? Can we afford life itself? Those questions were never asked as we destroyed the waters of our Nation, and they deserve no answers as we finally move to restore and renew them" (Simon 2019). The Senate and House shortly overrode the veto, and the bill was ultimately passed.

Since the passage of the CAA of 1970, the EPA has been required to develop national air quality standards, put forth motor vehicle emission standards, and establish emission standards for stationary sources. States were given the responsibility of creating emission reduction plans. In this act, Congress expanded enforcement authority by authorizing more comprehensive federal and state regulations to reduce emissions from both stationary (industrial) sources and mobile sources (e.g., automobiles).

Under this act, four major regulatory programs affecting stationary sources were initiated:

1. National Ambient Air Quality Standards (NAAQS), which pertain to six principal pollutants, called *criteria air pollutants*, that are considered harmful to public health and the environment: particulate matter, photochemical oxidants (including ozone), carbon monoxide, sulfur oxides, nitrogen oxides, and lead (EPA calls these pollutants criteria air pollutants because it sets NAAQS for them based on the latest scientific information regarding their effects on health or welfare)
2. State Implementation Plans, which are a collection of regulations and documents used by states, territories, or local air quality authorities to reduce air pollution in areas that do not meet NAAQS
3. New Source Performance Standards, which authorize the development of technology-based standards that apply to specific categories of stationary sources
4. National Emission Standards for Hazardous Air Pollutants, which are stationary source standards for hazardous air pollutants

Several events after the passage of the 1970 act led to further amendments. The oil embargo of 1973 and the energy crisis of the 1970s led to conflict over pollution control programs. Presidents Nixon, Ford, and Carter attempted to create a national energy policy, but all failed to achieve consensus. Ultimately, the Carter administration was forced to ease air pollution control requirements because of high inflation and increasing oil prices. Nonetheless, or despite these political barriers, as a result of a bipartisan effort led by Muskie, Baker, Robert Stafford (R-VT), Pete Domenici (R-NM), John Chafee (R-RI), and James Buckley (C-NY), the CAA was once again amended in 1977 (Clean Air Amendments of 1977). These amendments established more stringent standards to attain and maintain air quality control. These changes included the introduction of classification of attainment versus nonattainment areas (whether an area with concentrations of criteria pollutants is below or above the levels established by the NAAQS, respectively), the creation of the first federal permit program for new and modified stationary sources that would later be expanded to regulate industry, the definition of Prevention of Significant Deterioration, and the implementation of more stringent motor vehicle emissions standards.

Despite the effectiveness of the amendments in controlling air pollutant emissions, the administration of President Ronald Reagan sought to decrease government regulation, shift responsibilities to the states, and rely more on the private sector to achieve its ends in environmental policy and other policy arenas. Reagan administration officials argued that although the CAA had benefits in its initial years, the marginal utility of the act was diminishing, and they felt that each additional dollar spent on air pollution control would be inefficient (Augustine 2005). Although Reagan's overall efforts to deregulate environmental laws may have seemed to be a setback to air pollution control, they inspired zealous advocates for environmental protection. Following in Nixon's footsteps, President George H. W. Bush leveraged the American environmental consciousness, pledging to be "an environmental president" during the period in which the CAA was due to be amended. This promise was made possible with the replacement of Senate Majority Leader Robert Byrd (D-WV), a proponent of high-sulfur coal and midwestern utility companies, with Senator George Mitchell (D-ME), an ardent supporter of acid rain regulation.

In November 1988, Bush was elected in part on this platform, eventually culminating in the passage of the 1990 CAA amendments in the fall of that year. Congress extensively revised and expanded the CAA, providing the EPA even broader authority to implement and enforce regulations reducing air pollutant emissions (Clean Air Amendments of 1990). Under these amendments, the EPA was directed to a different approach to reducing toxic air pollutants. Instead of regulating air toxins one chemical at a time, the EPA began to identify larger and general categories of industrial sources for 187 listed toxic air pollutants and took steps to reduce pollution by requiring these sources to install controls or change production processes. For motor vehicles, the 1990 act required the EPA to issue a series of rules to reduce pollution from vehicle exhaust, refueling emissions, and evaporating gasoline. These regulations encouraged the development of new technologies and forced industrial facilities to use the most advanced control techniques available.

The 1990 act also introduced the Acid Rain Program under Title IV, the first nationwide cap and trade program, with the goal of reducing the emissions of sulfur dioxide (SO_2) and nitrogen oxides (NO_x) from power plants that fell under Title IV of the CAA. This highly successful program is an implementation of emissions trading that primarily targets coal-burning power plants, allowing them to buy and sell emission permits (called *allowances*) according to individual needs and costs. The undisputed success of the program in achieving significant emissions reductions in a cost-effective manner led to the deployment of this market-based cap and trade tool strategy to other environmental problems, namely, interstate air pollution transport, allowing states to be compensated for air pollution transported across state lines by the dynamics of air flow.

The CAA of 1990 also added the operating permit program under Title V for industrial and commercial sources that release pollutants into the air.

Operating permits include information on which pollutants are being released, how much may be released, and what kinds of steps the source's owner or operator is required to take to reduce the pollution. If requirements are not met, the EPA can take over issuing permits from states and tribes. Operating permits are especially useful for businesses covered by more than one part of the CAA because they consolidate information from all of the air pollution control requirements into a single, comprehensive document covering all aspects of the source's air pollution activities. The permit program simplifies and clarifies businesses' obligations for cleaning up air pollution and reduces administrative work.

Because the ozone layer, which protects humans from ultraviolet radiation, was gradually depleting in the stratosphere, in 1990 Congress added provisions to the CAA under Title VI to protect the stratospheric ozone layer. These provisions required the EPA to set up a program for phasing out production and use of ozone-destroying chemicals, including chlorofluorocarbons, halons, and methyl chloroform, and encouraging the development of "ozone-friendly" substitutes for the ozone-destroying chemicals.

These amendments granted the EPA important enforcement powers, allowing for easier penalization of a company for violating the CAA and increasing the range of civil and criminal sanctions available. If the EPA discovers that a violation has occurred, the agency can issue an order requiring the violator to comply, use EPA administrative authority to force payment of a penalty, or sue the violator in court.

One of the most important aspects of the 1990 amendments is that they directly give the public opportunities to contribute to the cleanup of pollution through required public hearings that determine how the law is carried out. The public is invited to hearings that are held across the country regarding major rules the EPA is working on. The public is also encouraged to participate in the development of state or tribal implementation plans and to share suggestions that are publicly viewed. Furthermore, this act allows the public to review industrial sources' air pollution permits and industry's air pollutant emissions. The 1990 act requires the EPA to publicly release information collected on air pollution data, including its monitoring and measuring of pollution released by industrial and commercial sources. Members of the public are even encouraged to work with the EPA, states, or tribes to take legal action against polluters.

Since 1992, the environment has continued to receive considerable attention. President Bill Clinton had much support from environmentalists when he selected as his running mate Senator Al Gore (D-TN), who had just published his provocative book *Earth in the Balance: Ecology and the Human Spirit* (Gore 1992). Although the Clinton administration was unable to make major progress in pollution control during its terms in office, it made some changes to enhance environmental protection, including the Safe Drinking Water Act Amendments of 1996, which created a new cost-effective approach to regulating contaminants in drinking water. Clinton also supported the controversial EPA clean air standards for ozone and fine particulates in 1997.

On October 20, 1999, a group of 19 private organizations (e.g., nonprofit organizations focused on environmental sustainability) filed a petition requesting that the EPA issue rules to regulate "greenhouse gas emissions from new motor vehicles under §202 of the CAA" (International Center for Technology Assessment 1999). Petitioners stated that 1998 was the "warmest year on record" and that carbon dioxide (CO_2), methane, nitrous oxide, and hydrofluorocarbons are "heat trapping greenhouse gases" that have significantly accelerated climate change. They referenced the Intergovernmental Panel on Climate Change's 1995 report (Intergovernmental Panel on Climate Change 1996), which stated that CO_2 was the "most important contributor to anthropogenic climate change." The petition further warned that "climate change will have serious adverse effects on human health and the environment."

After extensive public comment, the EPA denied the petition, stating that the EPA did not have authority under the CAA to issue mandatory regulations to address global climate change because it was not explicitly directed by Congress to do so and, therefore, greenhouse gases (GHGs) were not considered "air pollutants" under the CAA. The EPA further stated that it would not set standards for GHGs because there was uncertainty regarding the link between GHGs and global warming, the mandatory regulation was a piecemeal approach that would interfere with the president's more comprehensive approach, and it might hamper the president's ability to persuade developing countries to limit GHGs.

Ultimately, however, courts decided that the EPA has authority to regulate CO_2 and other GHGs as air pollutants under the CAA. The year 2007 brought revolutionary change to the CAA—the U.S. Supreme Court, in *Massachusetts v. EPA* (2007), ruled 5–4 in favor of Massachusetts and against the EPA that the EPA must regulate CO_2 emissions from motor vehicles if they are found to be endangering public health and welfare. Then, in 2009, for the first time, the EPA determined that emissions of CO_2 and other long-lived GHGs that build up in the atmosphere endanger the health and welfare of the public by causing climate change and ocean acidification. This determination would later be the basis for all EPA regulation of GHGs under Section 202(a) of the CAA (U.S. Environmental Protection Agency 2016a).

The Light-Duty Vehicle Greenhouse Gas Emission Standards and Corporate Average Fuel Economy Standards Rule set forth rules to further reduce GHG emissions and improve fuel economy for light-duty vehicles (any motor vehicle having a gross vehicle weight of no more than 8,500 pounds such as sedans and station wagons), light-duty trucks (trucks with a gross vehicle weight up to 8,500 pounds such as vans, minivans, sports utility vehicles, and pickup trucks), and medium-duty passenger vehicles (vehicles weighing less than 10,000 pounds and designed primarily for the transportation of persons) for models from 2012 to 2016 (U.S. Environmental Protection Agency 2016b). This rule provides for technological feasibility of complying with more stringent CO_2 emission reductions gradually, given the cost of compliance within such a period. The regulation is also flexible, allowing for banking and trading of credits, to allow for the decrease of total emissions through cap and trade policies. For example, credits are obtained when a manufacturer's models' average CO_2 emissions are less than the standard, and these credits can be used by the manufacturer itself or sold to another entity.

Although one of the greatest strengths in the CAA is the innovation of regulating air pollution on the basis of new scientific understandings of air pollution and its effects on health, this strategy is not without major pitfalls, one of which involves difficulty regulating GHGs under preestablished statutory language. Two other sections under the CAA, the Prevention of Significant Deterioration (PSD) and Title V, require permits for new and modified sources that emit 250 and 100 tons per year or more of any air pollutant, respectively. However, if applied to GHGs, millions of small sources such as small businesses, schools, and apartment buildings could be subject for the first time to the CAA's permitting requirement, a situation that would be extremely expensive and burdensome. Therefore, the EPA issued a "tailoring" rule to increase the threshold so that only sources with annual emissions of 75,000 or 100,000 tons or more of GHGs, depending on the circumstances, are subject to PSD and Title V. Even though the CAA states that PSD applies to major new and modified sources of "any air pollutant," petitioners such as the Coalition for Responsible Regulation argue that PSD cannot sensibly be applied to GHGs because PSD applies to only a subset of pollutants regulated as criteria pollutants under Sections 108 and 109 of the CAA (Carlson and Herzog 2014). Rather than designing a program to expand PSD to a more relevant set of pollutants for GHGs, the EPA chose to work within statutory language, which may not be applicable to GHG pollution.

Despite these many revisions over the past five decades, the CAA continues to evolve in accordance with the basic constitutional principles on which it was established in 1963: that the quality of the air impacts the welfare of U.S. citizens, which is protected under the Constitution. In this way, it continues to provide a constitutional basis for the development of air quality standards under evolving conditions and was prescient in its ability to protect the public's health.

Cleaner Air, Healthier Minds

It took the tragedy of suffocating, deadly smog—and the legislative savvy of Muskie and fellow politicians working to garner the political will to invest in cleaning our air—to bring about the CAA and related legislative victories. Through many decades of amendments and political agendas, the CAA has made tremendous strides toward accomplishing the goal of cleaner, safer air. New passenger vehicles are 98%–99% cleaner for most tailpipe pollutants than they were in the 1960s (U.S. Environmental Protection Agency 2018). Fuels are much cleaner—lead has been eliminated, and sulfur levels are more than 90% lower than they were prior to regulation. EPA standards have sparked technological innovations from industry (U.S. Environmental Protection Agency 2018). Moreover, despite their ever-increasing populations and increasing vehicular traffic, U.S. cities have had much improved air quality (Figure 5–3). Between 1990 and 2017, national concentrations of air pollutants improved 80% for lead, 77% for carbon monoxide, 88% for sulfur dioxide, 56% for nitrogen dioxide, and 22% for ozone (U.S. Environmental Protection Agency 2019). Fine particle concentrations improved 40%, and coarse particle concentrations improved 34% between 2000 and 2015 (U.S. Environmental Protection Agency 2019).

Reducing air pollution has led to significant improvements in pollutant exposure and therefore physical health (Table 5–1). For instance, CAA 1990 amendments resulted in a reduction in benzene of at least 80% in the highest-risk neighborhoods in Greater Houston, Texas (Ross et al. 2012). In 2010 alone, the CAA was estimated to have saved 160,000 lives, and the number of lives saved annually was expected to have topped 230,000 by 2020, according to a report released by the EPA in March 2017 (U.S. Environmental Protection Agency 2017a). Because of the reduction in fine particle and ozone pollution, the CAA was estimated to have led to the following disease reductions by 2020: 200,000 fewer heart attacks, 2.4 million fewer asthma attacks, 135,000 fewer hospital admissions, 120,000 fewer emergency department visits, and 17 million fewer lost workdays (U.S. Environmental Protection Agency 2017a). When expressed in economic terms, the report estimates that despite $65 billion spent by 2020 to comply with new regulations, the United States will reap more than $2 trillion as a result of the saving of life and health, improved environmental conditions, and increased economic welfare of Americans (U.S. Environmental Protection Agency 2011a; Ross et al. 2012).

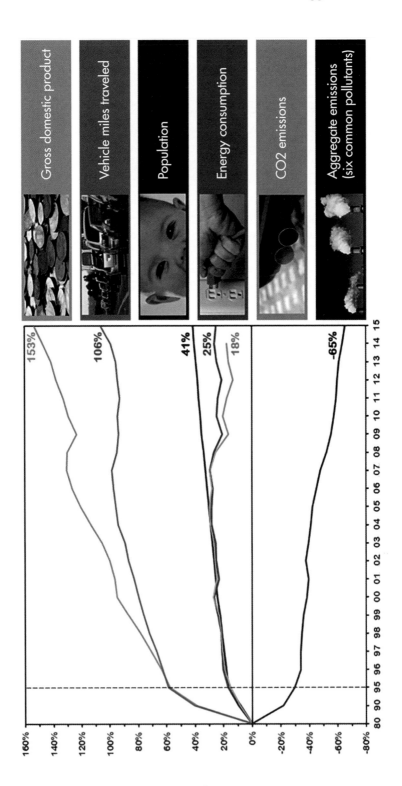

FIGURE 5–3. Comparison of growth areas and emissions, 1980–2015.

This graph shows decreases in U.S. air pollution emissions from transportation sources (e.g., cars, trucks, aircraft, construction and farm equipment) while the U.S. population and economic activity increased.

Source. U.S. Environmental Protection Agency: "Air Quality—National Summary." Washington, DC, U.S. Environmental Protection Agency, 2016a. Available at: www.epa.gov/air-trends/air-quality-national-summary. Accessed February 8, 2022. Public domain.

TABLE 5–1. Prevention of adverse outcomes attributable to the 1990 Clean Air Act Amendments

	Reductions (in cases)	
Adverse outcome	**2010**	**2020**
Adult mortality[a]	160,000	230,000
Infant mortality[a]	230	280
Mortality[b]	4300	7100
Chronic bronchitis	54,000	75,000
Heart disease (acute myocardial infarction)	130,000	200,000
Asthma exacerbation	1,700,000	2,400,000
Emergency room visits	86,000	120,000
Lost school days	3,200,000	5,400,000
Lost work days	13,000,000	17,000,000

[a]Lower mortality is due to reduced levels of fine particles.
[b]Lower mortality is due to reduced levels of ozone.

Source. Adapted from U.S. Environmental Protection Agency (2011b).

The effects of the CAA on mental health are both direct and indirect. Improving physical health, especially respiratory health, indirectly but significantly affects mental health. Several studies have shown an association between chronic respiratory problems and mood and anxiety disorders. Individuals with asthma have twice the risk of developing mood and anxiety disorders as individuals without asthma (Rosenkranz and Davidson 2009), and patients with severe chronic obstructive pulmonary disease (COPD) have a 2.5 times greater risk of depression than those without COPD (van Manen et al. 2002).

A direct impact of the CAA on mental health is the benefits from the reduction of lead pollution. Since the phaseout of lead-based gasoline by the EPA under the CAA, children's blood lead levels have continuously declined in the United States. In fact, this decrease in blood lead concentration strongly correlates with the decline in total lead used per year in gasoline. Children are extraordinarily vulnerable to the adverse health effects of lead poisoning. Physical health effects of lead poisoning include anemia, hypertension, renal impairment, and immunotoxicity (Abadin 2007). In addition, toxic accumulation of lead causes long-term neurodevelopmental problems, including learning disabilities, developmental delays, decreases in IQ scores, and reduced educational attainment. High levels of lead also lead to behavioral problems and antisocial behavior (Bellinger 2008). Blood lead levels of 10–20 µg/dL have been reliably associated with cognitive impairment and behavioral problems such as ADHD that may not manifest until school age (Wang et al. 2008). Cognitive deficits from lead can persist throughout childhood and beyond adolescence. The impact of the CAA on reducing lead emissions has been a huge step forward in decreasing lead toxicity, preventing 10.4 million lost IQ points in children as a result of lead exposure in 1990 alone (U.S. Environmental Protection Agency 2017c).

The CAA's effects on decreasing air pollutants has had impacts on other neurodevelopmental and neurocognitive disorders as well (Hertz-Picciotto et al. 2018; Peters et al. 2019). Researchers have found strong associations between autism and exposure to traffic-related air pollutants regulated by the CAA, as well as regional measures of particulate matter with diameters of 2.5 µm and smaller ($PM_{2.5}$), particulate matter with diameters of 10 µm and smaller (PM_{10}), and nitrogen dioxide (NO_2) (Fu et al. 2019). The magnitude of these associations was most pronounced during late gestation and early life. Autistic children were three times as likely to have been exposed during the first year of life to higher modeled traffic-related air pollution compared with typically developing control subjects. Exposure to traffic-related air pollution during pregnancy was also associated with autism to similar degrees (Volk et al. 2013).

Multiple studies have also linked air pollution to cognitive decline and increased incidence of Parkinson's disease and Alzheimer's disease (Chen et al. 2017; Fu et al. 2019; Oudin et al. 2016; Peters et al. 2019; Tzivian et al. 2016). One study showed that living close to heavy traffic was associated with a higher incidence of dementia (Chen et al. 2017). In this population-based cohort study of 243,611 incident cases of dementia, 7%–11% of dementia cases in those who lived near major roads were attributed to traffic exposure. The authors also found that both NO_2 and $PM_{2.5}$ were positively associated with dementia, suggesting that living near major roads may substantially increase an individual's exposure to traffic-related air pollution and thereby increase the risk for developing dementia. A systematic review of 26 studies found adverse effects of air pollution exposure on selected cognitive or psychomotor functions. For example, NO_2 exposure was linked to impaired working memory, general cognitive functions, and psychomotor functions. $PM_{2.5}$ exposure was linked to difficulties in working memory, short-term memory, attention, processing speed, and fine motor function (Lopuszanska and Samardakiewicz 2020).

Air pollution exposure has also been associated with depression. Studies in South Korea and the United States have shown that increases in pollutants, including PM_{10}, $PM_{2.5}$, NO_2, and ozone, are associated with increased risk of depressive symptoms and depression onset (Kioumourtzoglou et al. 2017; Lim et al. 2012; Power et al. 2015). Each 5 $\mu g/m^3$ increase in $PM_{2.5}$ has been associated with a 16% increase in depressive symptoms after adjusting for socioeconomic status (Pun et al. 2017). A meta-analysis showed that a 10 $\mu g/m^3$ increase in long-term exposure to $PM_{2.5}$ was associated with an 18% increased risk of depression (Liu et al. 2021). Studies have also found that higher concentrations of air pollutants are associated with increased psychiatric medication usage (Vert et al. 2017) and increased risk of emergency department visits for depressive episodes (Cho et al. 2014; Szyszkowicz 2007).

A recent study involving the analysis of large population data sets from the United States and Denmark suggested that there may be a strong link between exposure to environmental pollution and other mental illnesses, including bipolar disorder (Khan et al. 2019). Khan et al. analyzed information held in a U.S. health insurance database of 151 million individuals on a county level. Analyses in Denmark involved much smaller areas, just over one-quarter of a mile. In both countries, bipolar disorder risk was consistently associated with worse air quality. In the United States, counties with the worst air quality had a 27% increase in the prevalence of bipolar disorder. Similarly, in Denmark, there was a 29% increase in the incidence of bipolar disorder among people in areas with the worst air quality. These studies have been largely cross-sectional, and further investigation of the mechanisms linking air pollution and mental illnesses is needed.

In addition, numerous studies have found that high exposure to air pollutants is significantly associated with an increased risk of death by suicide. Studies conducted in South Korea, the United States, and China all found a strong association between short-term exposure to air pollutants (including PM_{10}, $PM_{2.5}$, and NO_2) and risk of suicide death (Bakian et al. 2015; Kim et al. 2010; Lin et al. 2016). On the basis of these results, Bakian and colleagues noted that there is now convincing global evidence for the positive association between suicide risk and air pollution, which persists with geographical, meteorological, and cultural variation (Bakian et al. 2015).

This significantly increased likelihood for suicide death was shown again more recently, this time in association with long-term exposure to air pollution (Min et al. 2018). A study including 265,749 adults in South Korea found that increases in long-term exposure to PM_{10} of 7.5 µg/m^3, NO_2 of 11.8 ppb, and SO_2 of 0.8 ppb were significantly associated with increased rates of suicide death of 309%, 33%, and 15% for each respective air pollutant. Therefore, it stands to reason that through strict policies regulating air pollutants, the CAA has had a major positive impact not only on physical health but also on mental health.

Various mechanisms have been proposed to explain the observed association between air pollution and mental health. Exposure to ambient particles and gaseous pollutants activates proinflammatory cytokines, leading to systemic and neuronal inflammation and subsequent oxidative stress, both systemically and in the brain (Calderón-Garcidueñas et al. 2010). There is also evidence that air pollutants may alter brain structure. Exposure to elevated levels of $PM_{2.5}$ was associated with smaller total cerebral brain volume, a marker of age-associated brain atrophy, and with higher odds of covert brain infarcts (Wilker et al. 2015). A prospective study of 1,403 community-dwelling older women without dementia showed a significant association between $PM_{2.5}$ exposure and white matter loss even after controlling for known risk factors (Chen et al. 2015). Moreover, postmortem studies have also shown the presence of abundant nanoparticles that precisely match airborne particulate matter in the human brain in those exposed to high air pollution (Maher et al. 2016). These studies, detailing the biological pathways of brain damage by air pollution, depicting structural deterioration in the brain, and demonstrating evidence of air pollutant particles in brains, suggest that organic brain damage may directly explain part of the link between air pollution and mental illness.

Under the 1990 CAA amendments, the Acid Rain Program achieved major success in significantly eliminating acid rain through reducing NO_x and SO_2. The program's reduction in acid rain has also led to improved mental health through improving visibility by reducing haze. Haze is created when sunlight is absorbed and blocked by many tiny pollution particles in the atmosphere and becomes absorbed and blocked by pollutants, resulting in reduced clarity and color in what we see. Mandated by Congress, the Regional Haze Program was established to further improve visibility in national parks and wilderness areas. As a result of this program, in eastern parks and wilderness areas (including areas such as Shenandoah National Park, Virginia, and Okefenokee National Wildlife Refuge, Georgia), the average visual range (the distance a visitor can see) has improved from 50 miles in 2000 to 70 miles in 2015 (U.S. Environmental Protection Agency 2016c). In western parks and wilderness areas (including areas such as Arches National Park, Utah, and John Muir Wilderness, California), the average visual range has improved from 90 miles to 120 miles over the same period (U.S. Environmental Protection Agency 2016c). Unfortunately, the increasingly severe annual wildfires as a result of climate change are now reversing this process. The National Park Service showed that during August 2021, the visibility in Rocky Mountain National Park remained less than 50 miles (Finley 2021).

Visibility of nature and landscapes can increase positive emotional states, including feelings of affection, friendliness, playfulness, and elation (Ulrich 1979, 1981). The CAA's achievement in reducing air pollution has affected air quality, the enjoyment of green and other natural spaces, and our ability to visibly appreciate our environment, all of which have positively contributed to the mental health of our society. In fact, perceived air pollution has been shown to be significantly associated with reduced subjective well-being (Li et al. 2018; Sun et al. 2018).

Progress on the Bumpy Road to Cleaner Air

Despite the great successes in reducing air pollutants for the past few decades, much more needs to be done to eliminate the danger to public health from air pollution—most prominently GHG emissions, the main drivers of climate change. Carbon dioxide accounts for most of the nation's GHG emissions and most of the increase since 1990. From 1990 to 2014, GHG emissions caused by human activities increased by 7%, and emissions have continued to rise since (U.S. Environmental Protection Agency 2017b). In fact, America's CO_2 emissions rose by 3.4% in 2018 (Rhodium Group 2019), the biggest increase in 8 years, occurring in the context of a loosening of policies limiting GHG emissions under the administration of President Donald J. Trump. A 2022 report from the World Meteorological Organization highlights the rapid advancement of climate change and necessitates a rapid move toward more stringent regulation of GHG emissions (World Meteorological Organization 2022).

In 2015, President Barack Obama finalized the Clean Power Plan, a signature climate measure designed to reduce GHG pollution from power plants to 32% below 2005 levels by 2030 (Friedman and Plumer 2017). President Trump viewed these EPA regulations as overly burdensome to the fossil fuel industry and proposed a rollback of this plan, lowering GHGs by only 0.7%–1.5% rather than 32% (Davenport and Friedman 2018). In addition to weakening these key climate regulations, on June 1, 2017, President Trump withdrew the United States from the Paris Agreement (Plumber 2017), a voluntary accord under which nearly every country in the world had agreed to reduce emissions. Trump believed that joint global action on climate change was antagonistic to his "America First" message and could be harmful to the economy (Ellis 2017), a perspective that did not incorporate the costs of GHG impacts. The decision to leave the Paris Agreement may have encouraged other countries, especially poorer countries, to do the same, creating an even bigger setback to years of hard-won progress on climate change. However, renewed hope emerged when President Joseph R. Biden rejoined the Paris Agreement with a goal to cut GHGs by 50% from 2005 levels by 2030.

The Trump administration also loosened regulations regarding the release of methane into the atmosphere. Methane is a potent GHG—25 times more powerful than CO_2 in trapping heat in the atmosphere (Yvon-Durocher et al. 2014). It is emitted from landfills and coal-fired power plants, burned as part of oil drilling operations, and routinely leaked into the atmosphere from faulty oil and gas wells. On June 30, 2021, President Biden signed a bill repealing a Trump era rule that rolled back regulations on methane emissions.

The GHGs from human activities that are the bulk of air pollution have been the most significant direct driver of observed climate change since the mid-twentieth century. We must therefore consider how air pollution under the CAA should be regulated to minimize climate change–related health impacts. From 1990 to 2015, the total warming effect from human-generated GHGs increased by 37% (U.S. Environmental Protection Agency 2017b), and that associated with CO_2 alone increased by 30%. Additionally, a growing body of research suggests that unless humanity takes forceful action to curb the GHG emissions that drive climate change, a host of serious climate-related disruptions will affect virtually every area of the globe. For instance, some tropical coastal areas of the planet, such as the Atlantic coast of South and Central America, could be hit by as many as six crises at a time by 2100 (Mora et al. 2018; Schwartz 2018). GHG emissions exacerbate such crises by warming the atmosphere, with a wide array of effects, including, but certainly not limited to, increasing frequency and severity (and therefore destructiveness) of storms, melting glaciers and sea level rise, increasing intensity and frequency of heat waves, and increasing drought in places that are not normally dry, "ripening conditions for wildfires and heat waves" (Mora et al. 2018, p. 1062; Schwartz 2018). The potential for widespread trauma in populations and subsequent mental health effects from such consequences is obvious, and there has been increasing attention on studying and documenting the mental health effects in scientific research.

Although climate change's potential for devastating effects on physical health have been recognized for decades, the impacts of climate change on mental health have been gaining more attention recently. The Fourth National Climate Assessment by the U.S. Global Change Research Program, which is a nonpartisan scientific committee that is mandated to produce a report to Congress and the president on climate change's consequences every 4 years, detailed the mental health consequences of both short- and long-term climate change–related events in 2018 (U.S. Global Change Research Program 2018). Mental health consequences of climate change range from minimal stress and distress symptoms to clinical disorders, such as anxiety, depression, PTSD, and suicidality. These impacts can occur through rising temperatures, environmental disasters, social disruption, and other social and environmental stressors.

Growing evidence has demonstrated that the rising temperatures that result from climate change increase suicidality (Walrath 2019). Several studies found that as temperatures climbed over the course of decades in the United States and Mexico, suicide rates also increased by 0.7% and 2.1%, respectively (Burke et al. 2018). Another study showed that temperature variability caused more than 60% of suicide variance in Finland (Helama et al. 2013). In the same study, a positive correlation between temperatures and suicide rates from 1751 (when statistical authorities began documenting suicides in the country) to 1990 (when a national suicide prevention program was put into place) was documented in Finland (Helama et al. 2013). Furthermore, suicide rates in Greece correlated more significantly with temperature than with unemployment (Fountoulakis et al. 2016b). One 2016 study of 29 European countries over a 13-year period showed that climatic variables were consistently a better predictor of suicide than socioeconomic factors (Fountoulakis et al. 2016a).

Environmental disasters caused by climate change also have devastating impacts on mental health. A meta-analysis of data on the relationship between disasters and mental illnesses found that 7%–40% of all subjects exposed to an environmental disaster showed some form of psychopathology (Clayton et al. 2017), the highest prevalence being acute traumatic stress immediately after a disaster. Other acute psychopathologies included phobias, somatic symptoms, alcohol use disorder, depression, and increased drug use. Although most people's acute symptoms of trauma and shock are reduced after conditions of security have been restored in a disaster area, many people develop PTSD, depression, generalized anxiety, and suicidality. Among a sample of people living in areas affected by Hurricane Katrina (in and around New Orleans, Louisiana, in 2005), suicide and suicidal ideation more than doubled, one in six people met diagnostic criteria for PTSD, and 49% of people living in an affected area developed anxiety and depression (Clayton et al. 2017). Environmental disasters are also associated with an increase in violence toward women and children. After Katrina, there were 47 reported cases of sexual assault; 93.2% of the victims were women, and 13.6% of the victims were age 14 or younger (National Sexual Violence Resource Center 2006). These disasters may also lead to personal losses and social disruption, which have been shown to compound PTSD symptoms (Bryant et al. 2017).

Climate change has also been shown to cause social disruption, which leads to adverse effects on mental health, especially among vulnerable communities such as Indigenous communities. The Inuit populations in circumpolar Canada, whose land is part of their social and cultural identity, have been undergoing increasing family stress, substance use, and suicidal ideation because of changes in snow and ice patterns (Willox et al. 2013). Members of the United Houma Nation in southern Louisiana, whose cultural traditions rely on the land, feel disconnected from ancestral land because of pollution and its destructive effects on the environment (Billiot 2017).

Although the CAA has positively affected mental health, the climate change that results from air pollution continues to pose major risks to mental health. New policies regulating air pollution could strongly affect mental health by specifically targeting the GHGs that are causing these disruptions and may currently represent the single largest air pollution–related threat to physical and mental health in the United States and globally. The evolution of the CAA amendments has led to the incorporation of GHGs as air pollutants because new scientific evidence shows that GHGs are the main drivers of anthropogenic climate change and that climate change is endangering public health and welfare. Therefore, the CAA presents a legal opportunity to reduce global warming emissions and to protect Americans' health. In fact, the current infrastructure-related legislative proposals under the Biden administration may represent by far the largest and most serious commitment of the federal government addressing climate change.

The CAA's success and improvements over the past several decades were led by key political figures driven in large part by public opinion as citizens demanded the elimination of smog and visible air pollution. Today, we face the challenges of too-lax regulations on GHGs and pressure to roll back minimal advances. In addition, on June 30, 2022, the Supreme Court issued a ruling that severely limited the EPA's ability to regulate carbon emissions from power plants under the CAA (*West Virginia v. Environmental Protection Agency* 2022). With the current knowledge of the disastrous future impacts of climate change on mental health, we need to be outspoken and share this knowledge with each other and with politicians so that we can address the urgent threat of climate change. One of the most significant forces that promoted passage of the 1970 CAA amendments was the high percentage of Americans who thought that air and water pollution was a serious problem. Americans increasingly understand climate change is endangering their own lives (Kotcher et al. 2020). Just as the passage of the CAA was influenced by demands of the majority, regulations on GHGs also can and will need to be changed by voices of the American people. Similarly, mental health professionals, including psychiatrists, have an important role to play in speaking out and educating the public about the connection between climate change and mental health.

References

Abadin H: Toxicological Profile for Lead. Atlanta, GA, Agency for Toxic Substances and Disease Registry, 2007

Air Pollution Control Act of 1955, Pub. L. 84–159.

Augustine P: The Clean Air Act: A Chronology. Edited by Brill DC. Knoxville, TN, Baker Center Publications, 2005

Bakian AV, Huber RS, Coon H, et al: Acute air pollution exposure and risk of suicide completion. Am J Epidemiol 181(5):295–303, 2015 25673816

Bellinger DC: Very low lead exposures and children's neurodevelopment. Curr Opin Pediatr 20(2):172–177, 2008 18332714

Billings LG: Eulogy at a service in thanksgiving for the life of the Hon. Edmund Sixtus Muskie (reprinted in S Doc No 104-17, March 30, 1996

Billings LG: The founder. Lewiston, ME, Edmund S. Muskie Foundation, 2000. Available at: www.muskiefoundation.org/founder.html. Accessed May 13, 2022.

Billings LG: Edmund S. Muskie: a man with a vision. Maine Law Review 67(2):233–238, 2015

Billiot SM: How do environmental changes and shared cultural experiences impact the health of indigenous peoples in south Louisiana? Arts and Sciences Electronic Theses and Dissertations, 2017. Available at: https://openscholarship.wustl.edu/cgi/viewcontent.cgi?article=2102&context=art_sci_etds. Accessed February 8, 2022.

Bryant RA, Gallagher HC, Gibbs L, et al: Mental health and social networks after disaster. Am J Psychiatry 174(3):277–285, 2017 27838935

Burke M, González F, Baylis P, et al: Higher temperatures increase suicide rates in the United States and Mexico. Nat Clim Chang 8(8):723–729, 2018

Calderón-Garcidueñas L, Franco-Lira M, Henríquez-Roldán C, et al: Urban air pollution: influences on olfactory function and pathology in exposed children and young adults. Exp Toxicol Pathol 62(1):91–102, 2010 19297138

Carlson A, Herzog M: EPA greenhouse gas rules at stake in U.S. Supreme Court. Chicago, IL, American Bar Association, 2014. Available at: www.americanbar.org/groups/environment_energy_resources/publications/trends/2013–14/march-april-2014/epa_greenhouse_gas_rules_stake_us_supreme_court. Accessed February 8, 2022.

Chen H, Kwong JC, Copes R, et al: Living near major roads and the incidence of dementia, Parkinson's disease, and multiple sclerosis: a population-based cohort study. Lancet 389(10070):718–726, 2017 28063597

Chen JC, Wang X, Wellenius GA, et al: Ambient air pollution and neurotoxicity on brain structure: evidence from women's health initiative memory study. Ann Neurol 78(3):466–476, 2015 26075655

Cho J, Choi YJ, Suh M, et al: Air pollution as a risk factor for depressive episode in patients with cardiovascular disease, diabetes mellitus, or asthma. J Affect Disord 157:45–51, 2014 24581827

Clayton S, Manning C, Krygsman K, et al: Mental Health and Our Changing Climate: Impacts, Implications, and Guidance. Washington, DC, American Psychological Association, 2017

Clean Air Act of 1963, Pub. L. 88-206.

Clean Air Amendments of 1970, Pub. L. 91-604.

Clean Air Amendments of 1977, Pub. L. 95-95.

Clean Air Amendments of 1990, Pub. L. 101-549.

Congressional Record: National Air Quality Standards Act of 1970—Senate, September 21, 1970, p 32,900. Available at: http://abacus.bates.edu/muskie-archives/ajcr/1970/CAA%20ESM%20Opening.shtml. Accessed May 13, 2022.

Davenport C, Friedman L: How Trump is ensuring that greenhouse gas emissions will rise. The New York Times, November 26, 2018. Available at: www.nytimes.com/2018/11/26/climate/trump-greenhouse-gas-emissions.html. Accessed February 8, 2022.

Ellis J: The Paris climate deal: what you need to know. The New York Times, June 1, 2017. Available at: www.nytimes.com/2017/06/01/climate/paris-climate-change-guide.html. Accessed February 8, 2022.

ExplorePAhistory.com: The 1948 Donora smog historical marker. ExplorePA history.com, 2019. Available at: https://explorepahistory.com/hmarker.php?markerId=1-A-14D. Accessed February 8, 2022.

Finley B: Air in Colorado mountain parks and wilderness no longer fresh. The Denver Post, August 16, 2021. Available at: www.denverpost.com/2021/08/16/colorado-air-quality-national-parks-haze-ozone. Accessed February 8, 2022.

Fountoulakis KN, Chatzikosta I, Pastiadis K, et al: Relationship of suicide rates with climate and economic variables in Europe during 2000–2012. Ann Gen Psychiatry 15(1):19, 2016a 27508001

Fountoulakis KN, Savopoulos C, Zannis P, et al: Climate change but not unemployment explains the changing suicidality in Thessaloniki Greece (2000–2012). J Affect Disord 193:331–338, 2016b 26796233

Friedman L, Plumer B: E.P.A. announces repeal of major Obama-era carbon emissions rule. The New York Times, October 9, 2017. Available at: www.nytimes.com/2017/10/09/climate/clean-power-plan.html. Accessed February 8, 2022.

Fu P, Guo X, Cheung F, Yung K: The association between PM2.5 exposure and neurological disorders: a systematic review and meta-analysis. Sci Total Environ 655:1240–1248, 2019 30577116

Gerard D, Lave LB: Implementing technology-forcing policies: the 1970 Clean Air Act amendments and the introduction of advanced automotive emissions controls in the United States. Technol Forecast Soc Change 72(7):761–778, 2005

Goldstein JK: Edmund S. Muskie: the environmental leader and champion. Maine Law Review 67(2):225–232, 2015

Gore A: Earth in the Balance: Ecology and the Human Spirit. New York, Houghton Mifflin, 1992

Helama S, Holopainen J, Partonen T: Temperature-associated suicide mortality: contrasting roles of climatic warming and the suicide prevention program in Finland. Environ Health Prev Med 18(5):349–355, 2013 23382022

Hertz-Picciotto I, Schmidt RJ, Krakowiak P: Understanding environmental contributions to autism: Causal concepts and the state of science. Autism Res 11(4):554–586, 2018 29573218

History.com: Killer smog claims elderly victims. History.com, October 29, 1948. 2009. Available at: www.history.com/this-day-in-history/killer-smog-claims-elderly-victims. Accessed February 7, 2022.

Holmes D: The smog that strangled Stan Musial's hometown of Donora, Pennsylvania. Baseball Egg, 2012. Available at: https://baseballegg.com/2012/10/19/the-strange-tragic-story-of-stan-musials-hometown-donora-pennsylvania. Accessed February 8, 2022.

Hopey D: Museum remembers Donora's deadly 1948 smog. Pittsburgh Post-Gazette, October 21, 2008. Available at: https://old.post-gazette.com/pg/08295/921526-85.stm. Accessed February 8, 2022.

Intergovernmental Panel on Climate Change: IPCC Second Assessment: Climate Change 1995. A Report of the Intergovernmental Panel on Climate Change. Geneva, World Meteorological Organization, 1996. Available at: https://archive.ipcc.ch/pdf/climate-changes-1995/ipcc-2nd-assessment/2nd-assessment-en.pdf. Accessed February 8, 2022.

International Center for Technology Assessment: Petition for rulemaking and collateral relief seeking the regulation of greenhouse gas emissions from new motor vehicles under § 202 of the Clean Air Act. Washington, DC, Center for International Environmental Law, 1999. Available at: www.ciel.org/Publications/greenhouse_petition_EPA.pdf. Accessed February 8, 2022.

Ivel J: Donora, Pennsylvania smog event of 1948. Guelph, ON, Canada, University of Guelph, 2017. Available at: www.soe.uoguelph.ca/webfiles/gej/AQ2017/Ivel/index.html. Accessed August 28, 2021.

Kenworthy EW: Tough new clean-air bill passed by Senate, 73 to 0. New York Times, September 23, 1970. Available at: www.nytimes.com/1970/09/23/archives/tough-new-cleanair-bill-passed-by-senate-73-to-0-a-tough-cleanair.html. Accessed May 13, 2022.

Kiester EJr: A darkness in Donora. Smithsonian Magazine, November 1999. Available at: www.smithsonianmag.com/history/a-darkness-in-donora-174128118/. Accessed February 8, 2022.

Khan A, Plana-Ripoll O, Antonsen S, et al: Environmental pollution is associated with increased risk of psychiatric disorders in the US and Denmark. PLoS Biol 17(8):e3000353, 2019 31430271

Kim C, Jung SH, Kang DR, et al: Ambient particulate matter as a risk factor for suicide. Am J Psychiatry 167(9):1100–1107, 2010 20634364

Kioumourtzoglou M-A, Power MC, Hart JE, et al: The association between air pollution and onset of depression among middle-aged and older women. Am J Epidemiol 185(9):801–809, 2017 28369173

Kotcher J, Maibach E, Rosenthal S, et al: Americans increasingly understand that climate change harms human health. Yale Program on Climate Change Communication, June 16, 2020. Available at: https://climatecommunication.yale.edu/publications/climate-change-harms-human-health. Accessed June 15, 2002.

Li Y, Guan D, Tao S, et al: A review of air pollution impact on subjective well-being: survey versus visual psychophysics. J Clean Prod 184:959–968, 2018

Lim Y-H, Kim H, Kim JH, et al: Air pollution and symptoms of depression in elderly adults. Environ Health Perspect 120(7):1023–1028, 2012 22514209

Lin G-Z, Li L, Song Y-F, et al: The impact of ambient air pollution on suicide mortality: a case-crossover study in Guangzhou, China. Environ Health 15(1):90, 2016 27576574

Liu Q, Wang W, Gu X, et al: Association between particulate matter air pollution and risk of depression and suicide: a systematic review and meta-analysis. Environ Sci Pollut Res Int 28(8):9029–9049, 2021 33481201

Lopuszanska U, Samardakiewicz M: The relationship between air pollution and cognitive functions in children and adolescents: a systematic review. Cogn Behav Neurol 33(3):157–178, 2020 32889949

Lydersen K: Remembering the deadly Donora smog. In These Times, October 27, 2014. Available at: https://inthesetimes.com/article/donora-smog. Accessed February 8, 2022.

Maher BA, Ahmed IAM, Karloukovski V, et al: Magnetite pollution nanoparticles in the human brain. Proc Natl Acad Sci USA 113(39):10797–10801, 2016 27601646

Massachusetts v EPA, 549 US 497 (2007)

Min J-Y, Kim H-J, Min K-B: Long-term exposure to air pollution and the risk of suicide death: a population-based cohort study. Sci Total Environ 628–629:573–579, 2018 29454198

Mora C, Spirandelli D, Franklin EC, et al: Broad threat to humanity from cumulative climate hazards intensified by greenhouse gas emissions. Nature Climate Change 8(12):1062–1071, 2018

National Sexual Violence Resource Center: Hurricanes Katrina/Rita and sexual violence: report on database of sexual violence prevalence and incidence related to hurricanes Katrina and Rita. Harrisburg, PA, National Sexual Violence Resource Center, 2006. Available at: www.nsvrc.org/publications/nsvrc-publications/hurricanes-katrinarita-and-sexual-violence-report-database-sexual-vi. Accessed February 9, 2022.

Orford A: The Clean Air Act of 1963: postwar environmental politics and the debate over federal power. Hastings Environmental Law Journal 27(2):article 2, 2021

Oudin A, Forsberg B, Adolfsson AN, et al: Traffic-related air pollution and dementia incidence in northern Sweden: a longitudinal study. Environ Health Perspect 124(3):306–312, 2016 26305859

Peters R, Ee N, Peters J, et al: Air pollution and dementia: a systematic review. J Alzheimers Dis 70(s1):S145–S163, 2019 30775976

Plumber B: What to expect as U.S. leaves Paris climate accord. The New York Times, January 1, 2017. Available at: www.nytimes.com/2017/06/01/climate/us-paris-accord-what-happens-next.html. Accessed February 8, 2022.

Power MC, Kioumourtzoglou MA, Hart JE, et al: The relation between past exposure to fine particulate air pollution and prevalent anxiety: observational cohort study. BMJ 350:h1111, 2015 25810495

Pun VC, Manjourides J, Suh H: Association of ambient air pollution with depressive and anxiety symptoms in older adults: results from the NSHAP study. Environ Health Perspect 125(3):342–348, 2017 27517877

Rhodium Group: Preliminary US emissions estimates for 2018. New York, Rhodium Group, January 8, 2019. Available at: https://rhg.com/research/preliminary-us-emissions-estimates-for-2018/. Accessed February 8, 2022.

Rinde M: Richard Nixon and the rise of American environmentalism. Distillations, June 2, 2017. Available at: www.sciencehistory.org/distillations/richard-nixon-and-the-rise-of-american-environmentalism. Accessed February 8, 2022.

Rosenkranz MA, Davidson RJ: Affective neural circuitry and mind-body influences in asthma. Neuroimage 47(3):972–980, 2009 19465136

Ross K, Chmiel JF, Ferkol T: The impact of the Clean Air Act. J Pediatr 161(5):781–786, 2012 22920509

Schrenk HH, Mountin JW: Air Pollution in Donora, Pa.: Epidemiology of the Unusual Smog Episode of October 1948: Preliminary Report. Washington, DC, Federal Security Agency, Public Health Service, Bureau of State Services, Division of Industrial Hygiene, 1949

Schwartz J: "Like a terror movie": how climate change will cause more simultaneous disasters. The New York Times, November 11, 2018. Available at: www.nytimes.com/2018/11/19/climate/climate-disasters.html. Accessed February 8, 2022.

Simon E: The bipartisan beginnings of the Clean Water Act. New York, Waterkeeper Alliance, January 30, 2019. Available at: https://waterkeeper.org/news/bipartisan-beginnings-of-clean-water-act. Accessed May 13, 2022.

Sun X, Yang W, Sun T, Wang Y: Negative emotion under haze: an investigation based on the microblog and weather records of Tianjin, China. Int J Environ Res Public Health 16(1):86, 2018 30598015

Szyszkowicz M: Air pollution and emergency department visits for depression in Edmonton, Canada. Int J Occup Med Environ Health 20(3):241–245, 2007 17932013

Transcript of the president's State of the Union message to joint session of Congress. The New York Times, January 23, 1970. Available at: www.nytimes.com/1970/01/23/archives/transcript-of-the-presidents-state-of-the-union-message-to-joint.html. Accessed February 8, 2022.

Tzivian L, Dlugaj M, Winkler A, et al: Long-term air pollution and traffic noise exposures and mild cognitive impairment in older adults: a cross-sectional analysis of the Heinz Nixdorf Recall study. Environ Health Perspect 124(9):1361–1368, 2016 26863687

Ulrich RS: Visual landscapes and psychological well-being. Landscape Research 4(1):17–23, 1979

Ulrich RS: Natural versus urban scenes: some psychophysiological effects. Environ Behav 13(5):523–556, 1981

U.S. Environmental Protection Agency: The benefits and costs of the Clean Air Act from 1990 to 2020: summary report. Washington, DC, U.S. Environmental Protection Agency, 2011a. Available at: www.epa.gov/sites/default/files/2015-07/documents/summaryreport.pdf. Accessed February 9, 2022.

U.S. Environmental Protection Agency: Benefits and costs of the Clean Air Act 1990–2020, the Second Prospective Study. Washington, DC, U.S. Environmental Protection Agency, 2011b. Available at: www.epa.gov/clean-air-act-overview/benefits-and-costs-clean-air-act-1990-2020-second-prospective-study. Accessed June 15, 2022.

U.S. Environmental Protection Agency: Endangerment and cause or contribute findings for greenhouse gases under the Section 202(a) of the Clean Air Act. Washington, DC, U.S. Environmental Protection Agency, 2016a. Available at: www.epa.gov/ghgemissions/endangerment-and-cause-or-contribute-findings-greenhouse-gases-under-section-202a-clean. Accessed February 8, 2022.

U.S. Environmental Protection Agency: Light-duty vehicle greenhouse gas regulations and standards. Washington, DC, U.S. Environmental Protection Agency, 2016b. Available at: www.epa.gov/greenvehicles/light-duty-vehicle-greenhouse-gas-regulations-and-standards. Accessed February 8, 2022.

U.S. Environmental Protection Agency: Protecting our nation's treasured vistas. Washington, DC, U.S. Environmental Protection Agency, 2016c. Available at: https://epa.maps.arcgis.com/apps/Cascade/index.html?appid=e4dbe2263e1f49fb849af1c73a04e2f2. Accessed February 8, 2022.

U.S. Environmental Protection Agency: Benefits and costs of the Clean Air Act, 1970 to 1990—study design and summary of results. Washington, DC, U.S. Environmental Protection Agency, 2017a. Available at: www.epa.gov/clean-air-act-overview/benefits-and-costs-clean-air-act-1970-1990-study-design-and-summary-results. Accessed February 8, 2022.

U.S. Environmental Protection Agency: Benefits and costs of the Clean Air Act amendments of 1990, fact sheet. Washington, DC, U.S. Environmental Protection Agency, 2017b. Available at: www.epa.gov/sites/default/files/2015-07/documents/factsheet.pdf. Accessed February 8, 2022.

U.S. Environmental Protection Agency: Climate change indicators: greenhouse gases. Washington, DC, U.S. Environmental Protection Agency, 2017c. Available at: www.epa.gov/climate-indicators/greenhouse-gases. Accessed February 8, 2022.

U.S. Environmental Protection Agency: History of reducing air pollution from transportation in the United States. Washington, DC, U.S. Environmental Protection Agency, 2018. Available at: www.epa.gov/transportation-air-pollution-and-climate-change/accomplishments-and-success-air-pollution-transportation. Accessed February 8, 2022.

U.S. Environmental Protection Agency: Progress cleaning the air and improving people's health. Washington, DC, U.S. Environmental Protection Agency, 2019.

Available at: www.epa.gov/clean-air-act-overview/progress-cleaning-air-and-improving-peoples-health. Accessed February 8, 2022.

U.S. Global Change Research Program: Fourth National Climate Assessment. Washington, DC, U.S. Global Change Research Program, 2018. Available at: https://nca2018.globalchange.gov. Accessed February 8, 2022.

van Manen JG, Bindels PJ, Dekker FW, et al: Risk of depression in patients with chronic obstructive pulmonary disease and its determinants. Thorax 57(5):412–416, 2002 11978917

Vert C, Sánchez-Benavides G, Martínez D, et al: Effect of long-term exposure to air pollution on anxiety and depression in adults: a cross-sectional study. Int J Hyg Environ Health 220(6):1074–1080, 2017 28705430

Volk HE, Lurmann F, Penfold B, et al: Traffic-related air pollution, particulate matter, and autism. JAMA Psychiatry 70(1):71–77, 2013 23404082

Walrath R: Climate change isn't just frying the planet: it's fraying our nerves. Mother Jones, February 18, 2019. Available at: www.motherjones.com/environment/2019/02/climate-change-isnt-just-frying-the-planet-its-fraying-our-nerves. Accessed February 8, 2022.

Wang H-L, Chen X-T, Yang B, et al: Case-control study of blood lead levels and attention deficit hyperactivity disorder in Chinese children. Environ Health Perspect 116(10):1401–1406, 2008 18941585

West Virginia v Environmental Protection Agency, No 20-1530, 2022. Available at: www.supremecourt.gov/opinions/21pdf/20-1530_n758.pdf. Accessed June 30, 2022.

Wilker EH, Preis SR, Beiser AS, et al: Long-term exposure to fine particulate matter, residential proximity to major roads and measures of brain structure. Stroke 46(5):1161–1166, 2015 25908455

Willox AC, Harper SL, Ford JD, et al: Climate change and mental health: an exploratory case study from Rigolet, Nunatsiavut, Canada. Climate Change 121(2):255–270, 2013

World Meteorological Organization: WMO update: 50:50 chance of global temperature temporarily reaching 1.5 degrees C threshold in next five years. Geneva, Switzerland, World Meteorological Organization, May 9, 2022. Available at: https://public.wmo.int/en/media/press-release/wmo-update-5050-chance-of-global-temperature-temporarily-reaching-15°c-threshold. Accessed June 15, 2022.

Yvon-Durocher G, Allen AP, Bastviken D, et al: Methane fluxes show consistent temperature dependence across microbial to ecosystem scales. Nature 507(7493):488–491, 2014 24670769

6 | Still on the Road to Freedom

The Civil Rights Act of 1964

Daniel Neghassi, M.D.
Taiwo P. Alonge, M.D., M.P.H.

Separate But Equal: A Deadly Myth

In 1937, John McBride, a young Black man who lived in Fort Lauderdale, Florida, was shot by a group of white vigilantes rumored to be members of the Ku Klux Klan (KKK). At the time, in true Jim Crow fashion, Fort Lauderdale police officers and white vigilantes alike did everything in their power to uphold racial segregation. Police fined Black people for "loitering," and if they could not pay the fines, which was often the case, Black people would be arrested and used as convict labor. White vigilantes, who effectively served as police auxiliaries, terrorized Black people who ventured into the predominantly white downtown Fort Lauderdale area. Not infrequently, they would gather in large groups, hop in their vehicles with weapons in hand, and physically attack and murder Black people.

In the case of McBride, despite being shot in the abdomen, he did not die immediately and could have been saved if his injuries were tended to expeditiously. He was turned away from the only two hospitals in the city be-

133

cause of the color of his skin. Dr. Von D. Mizell, the first Black surgeon in the state of Florida, pleaded and eventually convinced Broward General Hospital to make space for McBride, although they would only offer him a bed in the rat-infested sanitarium (Dolen 2020). That was where McBride would eventually die: murdered by white vigilantes and having his emergency care upended by racial segregation in the hospital.

Stories like McBride's were, unfortunately, par for the course for Black people seeking medical care before the passage of the Civil Rights Act of 1964 (CRA). At best, white hospitals had few beds in separate "colored wards," where the treatment was several notches below the standard of care given to white patients under the very same roof. Injustices like these existed in every facet of life. Black people were systematically blocked from living in decent neighborhoods, and the schools they attended were wholly inadequate. The substandard conditions and the constant threat of violence took a serious toll—physically and mentally—on the health of Black Americans. In response to the constant assault on their humanity, Black people mobilized and fought for equal rights, giving rise to the civil rights movement in the mid-twentieth century. Some of the movement's goals and demands would be met by the CRA, which outlawed racial and other types of segregation in public spaces, employment, and other parts of society. The CRA would create the conditions for better mental health by paving the way for some improved opportunities for Black Americans and dampening the injustices perpetuated by a deeply segregated society.

The conditions that prompted the civil rights movement and, eventually, the CRA did not arise out of thin air. Following the freeing of enslaved Black people in the United States in the mid-1860s, Black Americans made modest political and economic gains during the brief period known as Reconstruction (Equal Justice Initiative 2020). There was even limited support from the federal government with the 1865 establishment of the Freedmen's Bureau, a short-lived agency that provided rations, shelter, education, and other aid to formerly enslaved people. Out of this era emerged clusters of tightly knit communal Black towns with thriving businesses and livelihoods, populated by Black intellectuals, politicians, and professionals. This is not to say the period was without hardship, however. Poverty and desolation among newly freed Black people were widespread.

Ultimately, it was not a priority for policy makers to support the Black community in this time of transition. Before the Freedmen's Bureau was dissolved in 1872, a sizable portion of its funding was shunted to aid former enslavers to make up for the loss of the uncompensated labor. Furthermore, after the contested 1876 presidential election, Reconstruction was terminated as part of the Compromise of 1877, a deal that allowed Republicans to hold onto the presidency in exchange for pulling the last of the troops out of former Confederate states (McGreevy 2021). In other words, progress for Black people was sold out for political stability.

With slavery no longer the dominant legal institution to propagate America's racial caste system, a new wave of anti-Black racism was birthed out of white resentment. America saw the formation of white supremacist hate groups such as the KKK. White mob violence targeted and destroyed numerous thriving Black communities that were built during Reconstruction. Powerful factions of both major political parties (e.g., Southern Democrats, Lily White Republicans) were created with the sole aim of developing new ways to legislate anti-Black white supremacy. Jim Crow laws emerged as the new institutional pillar upholding the racist social hierarchy, especially in the South. With Jim Crow in place, Black and white people were separated in every aspect of life, including housing, education, the workplace, and health care. The segregationist rules and practices were bolstered by the Supreme Court decision *Plessy v. Ferguson* (1896), which ruled that the "separate but equal" doctrine was constitutional.

A year after McBride's untimely death, Drs. Mizell and James F. Sistrunk cofounded Provident Hospital, a 15-bed hospital providing care to Black residents of south Florida. This was part of a nationwide effort by Black advocates who established hundreds of hospitals across the country to address the stark lack of access to health care within the Black community. Unfortunately, because of limited funding and staffing, patient rooms in Black hospitals in the Jim Crow South were overcrowded, so much so that the hallways, which doubled as overflow areas, were narrowed by patients' beds. Services provided at these hospitals simply could not meet the demands of the large populations they served.

Meanwhile, there was no shortage of adequately resourced white hospitals, exposing separate but equal as the myth that it was. One major source of disparities in funding was the Hospital Survey and Construction Act of 1946, or, as it is more commonly known, the Hill-Burton Act, which provided grants and loans to build health care facilities on the basis of a region's population and per capita income. This meant that wealthy—and therefore white—communities qualified for larger grants. By 1975, nearly one in three hospitals in the country was built with Hill-Burton funds. When the bill was being debated, Northern legislators argued for nondiscrimination requirements, but ultimately, they appeased Southerners and allowed for segregated facilities, provided that supposedly equitable services were available for all groups, which was obviously impossible in reality given its funding provisions. It was the only federal legislation in the twentieth century that codified separate but equal in the disbursement of federal funds (Largent 2018).

This is the context of the civil rights movement that pushed for and helped craft the CRA, a bill that would seek to undo separate but equal practices in many aspects of society. The battle for the recognition of Black people's humanity was fought visibly on the streets, as well as behind the scenes in the courtrooms and in the chambers of Congress. Many different threads to this story exist. In this chapter we highlight just a few of the pieces that came together to make this landmark legislation possible, how the law affected social determinants of mental health, and, in the end, how it fell short in righting the wrongs of the Jim Crow era. First, however, we explore one thread of this story: the life and legacy of one of the most influential civil rights activists, Ella Baker.

Ella Baker: Leveraging People Power

Today, in mainstream interpretations of Black history, stories about the civil rights movement are often simplistically told as victories of charismatic, usually male, individuals acting alone in the fight against segregation, culminating in the passage of the CRA and related legislation. In the process, collectivism, issues other than racial integration, and the women paramount to the success of the movement are left out. If there is one person whose story best encapsulates the truly community-based ethos of the civil rights era, the broader demands of the movement beyond desegregation and the CRA, and the crucial role of Black women, it is Ella Josephine Baker (Figure 6–1).

"Miss Ella Baker," as she was affectionately called, empowered those who felt powerless and elevated the voices of youth because she knew the key to the sustainability of any struggle would lie in their hands (Ransby 2003). As Harry Belafonte once said, "Baker worked with…all of the well-known civil rights leaders but most importantly the unknown people. Her life has always been devoted to helping ordinary people in struggle develop their own leadership potential" (Grant 1981). She was quick to criticize and rebuke individualistic leadership even if it meant going toe-to-toe with prominent leaders such as Rev. Martin Luther King Jr. or the national organizations she worked within, such as the National Association for the Advancement of Colored People (NAACP). Over her lifetime, Baker fought against segregation, sexism, police brutality, educational inequity, and poverty—issues she knew were interrelated. Her drive to organize and speak out on these issues was based on values shaped by her upbringing and early adult life.

Baker was born on December 13, 1903, in post-Reconstruction Norfolk, Virginia, and grew up in her mother's hometown in Littleton, North Carolina. She was brought up surrounded by resolute Black women, most notably her mother, Ann Ross Baker, and her grandmother, Josephine Elizabeth "Bet" Ross. Ella Baker saw her mother and other women take on key

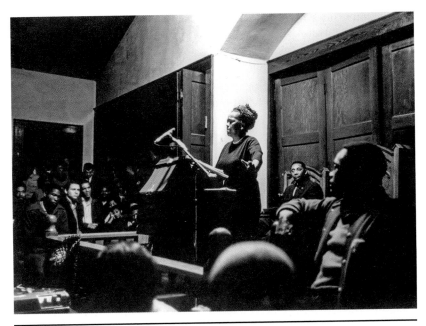

FIGURE 6–1. Ella Baker addresses a group from the podium, January 1964.
Source. George Ballis/TakeStock, TKS0820001, 1976.. Available at: http://takestockphotos.com/images/0820001.jpg. Accessed June 30, 2022. Used with permission.

leadership roles in the Black Baptist church. Bet Ross, who was formerly enslaved, would tell her grandchildren countless stories of the preemancipation times. She spoke not only of the hardships she experienced as an enslaved woman but also of the triumphs of her resistance and the preservation of her humanity. Ella Baker's grandparents owned a farm and engaged with other Black farmers in the community in cooperative arrangements such as buying goods together and sharing equipment. Through the guidance of her mother and grandmother, Ella Baker helped establish her perseverance and strong sense of community empowerment and mutual aid.

Ella Baker attended Shaw University, a Black Baptist college in Raleigh, North Carolina, where she often stirred up trouble as an activist. After graduating as valedictorian, she was offered several roles in education, the field that women were often expected to enter after college. Baker did not want to quell her fighting spirit by following the expected path, so she turned down the job offers in order to move to New York City. She was immediately drawn to the intellectual scene in Harlem, where she frequently discussed politics with journalist George Schuyler, activist Marvel Cooke, and many others. Although she struggled to find a job initially because of the Great Depression, she eventually found work at the Harlem Library organizing events on decolonization, class struggle, and anti-racism. In 1934, she was hired to coordinate an educational program called the Young People's Forum at the Harlem Library. This group was one of the first examples of Baker's keen understanding of intergenerational consciousness and the importance of empowering youth. In her work with the Young People's Forum, Baker was able to teach on her own nontraditional and uncaged terms.

Baker's economic and political perspectives were informed by debating politics with people with a range of ideologies, witnessing the extreme difficulty that many Black people faced during the Great Depression, and her sense of community empowerment from childhood. She believed that the relentless competition of capitalism led to the 1929 stock market crash and worsening economic inequality. This led her to become the national director for a new organization, the Young Negroes' Cooperative League, founded by Schuyler. The Young Negroes' Cooperative League advocated for the economic liberation of Black people, educated communities about alternative economic models, and helped establish cooperatives that prioritized investing in communities over individual profits. Baker also engaged in journalism and wrote about the plight of Black people in America—especially Black women—under the conditions of the Great Depression. In a piece she coauthored with Cooke, "The Bronx Slave Market," she chronicled the physically and mentally taxing conditions that Black women endured as maids for white people (Ransby 2003).

In the 1940s, Baker took her refined organizing talents to the NAACP, which fought for desegregation and economic justice primarily through lobbying and civil rights lawsuits (Figure 6–1). Baker's roles with the organization, initially as assistant field secretary and eventually as the national director of branches, required her to travel, usually to the South, where Black people faced the brunt of Jim Crow segregation. Baker worked tirelessly to organize ordinary people using her humanistic approach of self-empowerment and relationship building. She slept in people's homes, broke bread with them, and attended church with them. Baker always believed the NAACP could strengthen itself by decentralizing its leadership and establishing more local centers, insisting that the strength of the organization grew from the bottom up and not the top down (Ransby 2003).

Although women were central to the success of the NAACP, they were notably absent from senior leadership roles. Men remained the face of the highly bureaucratic organization, while fieldwork, disproportionately performed by women, carried risks of encounters with white vigilantes and hostile police officers. Although Baker was never arrested, she had some rough run-ins with law enforcement. Additionally, the Federal Bureau of Investigation (FBI), under its Counter Intelligence Program (COINTELPRO), closely surveilled her as well as countless other civil rights leaders, deeming them a threat to the status quo of a segregated America.

In 1946, still concerned with the NAACP's bureaucratic practices and its limiting of leadership to men, Baker resigned from the national office. The connections she formed from her field work kept her active as she continued to organize and give speeches to various NAACP branches. By the late 1940s and early 1950s, she found herself back in New York, tapped back into the political scene, and was eventually the first woman to be elected president of the New York City NAACP branch. Although she held the role for only a year, she managed to build coalitions that worked to desegregate schools and protest police brutality. These were two of many major issues that civil rights activists wanted local and national policy to address.

Desegregation of public services such as transportation was another such issue. In 1947, Baker had volunteered for the Journey of Reconciliation, an interracial group of activists riding on coach buses to push for desegregation, but was turned down because she was a woman. The Journey of Reconciliation was an inspiration for the successful Montgomery bus boycott, which was kicked off by Rosa Parks famously refusing to give up her seat at the front of the bus and ended after 381 days when the city's buses were finally desegregated in 1956. Civil rights leaders, including King, wanted to build on the momentum, organize more boycotts throughout the South, and bring continued national attention to the issue. Baker moved to Atlanta in 1958 to help King form what would become the Southern Christian Leadership Conference (SCLC). She was instrumental in shaping its agenda, although she faced frustrations similar to those she faced at the NAACP. Once again, Baker wanted to devote more resources to accomplishing the mission on the ground rather than supporting its charismatic male leaders (Elliott 1996).

Along the same lines, she saw the enactment of civil rights legislation as the start rather than the end of the struggle for freedom, knowing that a law's stated intent might be hampered or not even implemented at all. Instead, she wanted to create meaningful and sustainable change by organizing and supporting grassroots activism across the country to continually push for progress.

While serving as executive secretary for the SCLC, Baker saw an opportunity to support young emerging activists. In February 1960, a group of Black students from North Carolina Agricultural and Technical College organized a sit-in at the Woolworth's lunch counter in Greensboro, North Carolina, refusing to leave after being denied service. Recognizing their potential, Baker arranged a meeting with the leaders of the sit-in at her alma mater, Shaw University. At Baker's request, King agreed to have the SCLC financially support the gathering, hoping that they would form the student branch of his organization. However, Baker encouraged the students to consider starting their own organization with a group-centered leadership. The students were aligned with that approach and formed what would be known as the Student Nonviolent Coordinating Committee (SNCC, pronounced *snick*). Baker relished engaging with and teaching the students using the Socratic method and ensured that everyone's voice was heard. She tapped into her extensive network from her work as an NAACP field secretary to help support SNCC in their actions for years to come. Many of their activities were directed at voting rights, including Freedom Day in Hattiesburg, Mississippi, on January 22, 1964.

By this time, Congress was considering the bill that would become the CRA, and some hopeful activists thought they were in the final stages of the freedom struggle. In her address to the Hattiesburg demonstrators, Baker challenged this viewpoint, arguing that even if segregation were demolished and voting were accessible for all, "people cannot be free until...we recognize that in this country in a land of great plenty and great wealth, there are millions of people who go to bed hungry every night" (Baker 2006, p. 687). Contending that economic and racial justice are inextricably linked, she consistently pushed for her fellow activists to think broadly about the struggle for humanity and freedom. And because she connected with everyday people across the country, she knew how constant discrimination, poverty, hunger, and other traumatizing conditions harmed the collective psyche. Even though she knew abolishing segregation was inadequate, it was certainly a needed step toward freedom. The CRA aimed to be that step.

On the Way to Desegregation: Precedent and Protest

The work of civil rights activists was the impetus for the passage of the CRA. Nevertheless, the legislative actions and judicial decisions in the century prior to the CRA were also significant. The legal backdrop was a rollercoaster of progress and setbacks for civil rights. Three constitutional amendments and two civil rights acts were enacted in quick succession during Reconstruction to establish rights for formerly enslaved people who had recently been freed. The Thirteenth Amendment, enacted in 1865, abolished slavery and involuntary servitude, except as punishment for a criminal conviction. The Civil Rights Act of 1866 defined citizenship without regard to race or previous condition of slavery. It also gave all citizens the right to enter into contracts, own property, and benefit from laws. These provisions were further established by the Citizenship Clause and

Equal Protection Clause of the Fourteenth Amendment, ratified in 1868. The Fifteenth Amendment, adopted in 1870, prohibited the federal and state governments from denying the right to vote to U.S. citizens on the basis of race, color, or prior enslavement. The last of the major Reconstruction measures, the Civil Rights Act of 1875, prohibited racial discrimination in public transportation and public accommodation.

These laws, although important, were limited in scope and impact by loopholes and court decisions. For instance, the Fifteenth Amendment was rendered ineffective because many states used poll taxes and literacy tests to disenfranchise its Black would-be voters. Additionally, in a landmark 1883 decision, the Supreme Court took a narrow interpretation of these laws. Most notably, it ruled that the Equal Protection Clause of the Fourteenth Amendment could not be applied to private entities and that the Civil Rights Act of 1875 was unconstitutional. This was the legal precedent until the 1930s, when Supreme Court justices determined that the Interstate Commerce Clause gave Congress the authority to have more regulation over the private sector. This paved the way for future antidiscrimination legislation such as the CRA.

Another lawsuit decades later would give policy makers an even stronger legal foundation for the CRA. In 1962, less than 2 miles from the Greensboro Woolworth's lunch counter where the sit-ins took place, a Black Agricultural and Technical College student walked into a dental clinic with a painfully swollen mouth and high fever. The dentist, Dr. George Simkins Jr., one of the most highly regarded providers in town, quickly concluded that his patient needed oral surgery to prevent the abscessed tooth from making him septic. Simkins's first call was to the hospital down the block from his clinic, L. Richardson Memorial Hospital, a hospital for Black patients. Incredibly, the wait for an available bed was going to be at least 2 weeks. Simkins then turned to the two other hospitals in town, Moses H. Cone Memorial Hospital and Wesley Long Community Hospital. Both were operated by white people, and both had received federal Hill-Burton funds. Neither would admit his patient. Simkins applied for admitting privileges and, as a Black professional, was predictably denied at both institutions (Smith 2016). The injustices John McBride faced were still very much in play 25 years after his murder.

Simkins had experience with challenging the status quo. He had previously worked with NAACP Legal Defense Fund director-counsel Jack Greenberg on efforts to desegregate a local golf course, and he would later become the Greensboro chapter president. After facing challenges with getting his patient admitted to the hospital, he called Greenberg. Simkins gathered a group of plaintiffs consisting of medical professionals and patients. They filed a lawsuit, asserting that the racist policies of Cone Memorial and Wesley Long were violating their rights under the Equal Protection Clause. As required by law, the Legal Defense Fund's lawyers notified the U.S. Department of Justice (DOJ) that this suit was challenging the constitutionality of a federal statute, namely, the Hill-Burton Act.

This was nothing short of a political gift to President John F. Kennedy and his younger brother, Attorney General (AG) Robert F. Kennedy, who were looking to advance the civil rights platform without making too many waves. Nearly a decade earlier, the Supreme Court, in *Brown v. Board of Education of Topeka*, ended legal segregation in public schools, but that ruling did not apply to private entities. If the courts struck down the separate but equal provision for federally funded hospitals, the administration could then insist that bills establishing nondiscrimination requirements for federally funded private facilities were simply following established law. Although it was unprecedented for the DOJ to admit that a federal law is unconstitutional, AG Kennedy quietly submitted a memo in support of Simkins and his coplaintiffs (Largent 2018).

The district court sided with the hospitals, but the Fourth Circuit Court reversed it on appeal. The appellate justices ruled that as recipients of substantial federal funds, the hospitals were essentially carrying out a government function and therefore had a duty to not violate constitutional rights. The Supreme Court declined to hear *Simkins v. Cone* on appeal, so the appellate court decision was final. The separate but equal provision of the Hill-Burton Act was found unconstitutional, and the ruling built a legal foundation for Title VI, the part of the CRA that would dictate rules for nondiscrimination in federally funded programs.

Although the evolving case law was critical to quietly making progress on civil rights legislation, other battles were fought out in the open and put public pressure on lawmakers to take action. One of the most prominent examples was the Freedom Rides of 1961. Like the Journey of Reconciliation that came before them, the Freedom Rides were organized by the Congress of Racial Equality (CORE) and were launched to test compliance with a number of landmark Supreme Court decisions that barred segregation in interstate travel. In defiance of these rulings, waiting rooms at bus depots were still segregated, and Black passengers were forced to sit in the back of coach buses. Despite pressure from activists, the Kennedy administration hesitated to enforce these rulings through the Interstate Commerce Commission (ICC), giving credence to Baker's perspective that legal victories were not sufficient. The first Freedom Ride consisted of two buses leaving Washington, D.C., on May 4, 1961, with a planned route through the South. The original riders were an interracial group of young men and women trained in nonviolence tactics and included future SNCC chairperson and future 17-term U.S. Representative John Lewis (Figure 6–2).

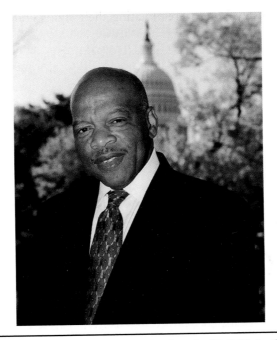

FIGURE 6–2. **Representative John Lewis (D-GA), in Congress 1987–2020.**

Source. Congress.gov. Public domain.

In Alabama, the Freedom Riders encountered extreme violence from Klansmen, who bombed and destroyed the lead bus and brutalized riders from the second bus. The Birmingham police commissioner had enabled the KKK violence and ensured that the local police did not intervene. The FBI also did not show up, despite having an informant who notified them of the KKK's plans. After the hostilities in Alabama, most of the original riders were unable to continue. AG Kennedy, who was assigned by the president to take a lead role in civil rights, suggested a "cooling off period" (Bagwell 1987). However, the Freedom Riders refused to stop. Even though they knew they risked more violence and even death, activists believed that stopping so early would send a message that future demonstrations could easily be shut down with violence. Members from SNCC, CORE, and the SCLC organized more rides, mostly converging in Jackson, Mississippi.

AG Kennedy had made a deal with Mississippi authorities. They could enforce the segregationist laws as long as they protected the riders from bloodshed. After police arrested the first set of riders to arrive in Jackson, organizers sent more Freedom Rides into the city. By the end of the summer, 300 participants were arrested, many of whom were sent to maximum security prison. As the racial conflict continued to receive national and even international headlines, political pressure mounted. In response, AG Kennedy asked the ICC to create new interstate travel regulations prohibiting segregation. The ICC complied in November 1961, scoring a major victory for the movement.

Over the years, law enforcement systemically ignored, enabled, or perpetuated violence against protesters who assembled peacefully (Hassett-Walker 2021). In addition to striving for desegregation, civil rights activists also demanded a stop to the police brutality that upheld the systems of segregation that was seen with the Freedom Rides and in countless other examples. They wanted the Kennedy administration to use executive power to enforce the laws already on the books (i.e., previous civil rights acts and the Equal Protection Clause of the Fourteenth Amendment) in order to address police brutality. They maintained that the DOJ could have filed an injunction against police departments that refused to allow Black Americans the right to peacefully protest. Cops who violated the injunction would have been sentenced to jail. However, the Kennedys were not willing to take what they saw as a federal overstep. Moreover, by their calculations, any legislation that included protections against police brutality would have little chance of passing Congress. When a House subcommittee was considering such a proposal in a section of the new civil rights bill, AG Kennedy went to the subcommittee to testify against that proposal. The section on police brutality never made it into the bill (Zinn 1965).

Amid ongoing organizing from civil rights groups and violent retaliation from white supremacists, President Kennedy introduced the civil rights bill in June 1963. After his assassination in November of that year, it was initially unclear how much incoming President Lyndon B. Johnson would accomplish in the realm of civil rights and with this bill in particular. Political aides advised the new president to table the divisive issue amid having to deal with numerous other challenges, not least of all the investigation into Kennedy's assassination. Instead, Johnson turned the civil rights bill into his legislative priority. As a former Senate majority leader, President Johnson demonstrated masterful political maneuvering to push the bill through Congress. He cut deals with key legislators, ensured that the bill moved through committees, and, along the way, publicly shamed Republicans, the so-called "party of Lincoln," for obstructing civil rights if they did not support the bill (O'Donnell 2014).

The bill passed the House after a number of amendments strengthened it. One of the most impactful of these amendments, submitted by Representative Howard Smith, expanded the list of classes protected against employment discrimination to include sex. Although a popular theory suggests that Smith, a Southern segregationist, was trying to tank the entire bill, the

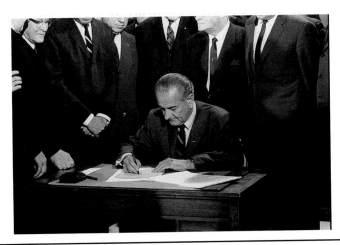

FIGURE 6-3. **President Lyndon B. Johnson signs the 1968 Civil Rights Bill.**
Source. Warren K. Leffler. Available from Library of Congress Prints and Photographs Division LC-U9- 18985-18A [P&P]. Available at https://loc.gov/resource/ppmsca.03196. Accessed: June 30, 2022.

amendment was, in fact, the result of effective lobbying by women's rights advocates (Onion 2020). When the bill went to the Senate for consideration, a coalition of mainly Southern Democrats launched a filibuster in an attempt to obstruct the bill. This tactic was used disproportionately by segregationists to block civil rights legislation in the twentieth century (Beauchamp 2021). In order to overcome the obstruction, Senate leaders on both sides of the aisle reworked some of the bill's language and enlisted sufficient support to break the record-breaking, 60-day-long filibuster. Just over a year after the bill was first introduced, the Senate version was sent back to the House, where it managed to pass without any further modification. That same night, July 2, 1964, President Johnson signed the bill into law (Figure 6–3).

Civil Rights Act of 1964

The CRA (Civil Rights Act of 1964) was one of a series of laws that aimed to address racial and other forms of discrimination. One of the more substantive sections of the law, Title II, pertains to public accommodations engaged in interstate commerce: hotels, restaurants, gas stations, theaters, stadiums, and similar establishments. It states, "All persons shall be entitled to the full and equal enjoyment of the goods, services, facilities, and privileges, advantages, and accommodations of any place of public accommodation...without discrimination or segregation on the ground of race, color, religion, or national origin." It gives the AG the responsibility to investigate and bring civil action against establishments that demonstrate a pattern or practice of discrimination or segregation.

Titles III and IV require desegregation in public facilities and in public education, respectively. Together, these two titles cover all facilities that are owned or run by government entities. Under Title III, public facilities cannot deny anyone equal use of the facility on account of race, color, religion, or national origin. This section of the law also directs the AG to take legal action on behalf of individuals who file a complaint of discrimination in public facilities and are unable to pursue the lawsuit on their own. Similarly, under Title IV, the AG may bring charges on behalf of students or their parents who have been subject to ongoing segregation in public schools. This applies to elementary schools up through higher education as well as technical or vocational programs that are operated by or funded predominantly by the government. Furthermore, the secretary of education was granted the authority to provide technical assistance to school districts to implement a plan to desegregate.

Title VI prohibits programs receiving federal assistance from discriminating against people on the basis of race, color, or national origin. Programs subject to Title VI regulations include schools, health care facilities, welfare agencies, and nonprofit grant recipients, among many others. Although it was not written into the law, the courts later determined that violations of Title VI can be intentional or can be the unintended result of practices that have a disparate impact on one population compared with another (Chambers 2008).

Title VII relates to discrimination within employment practices. Although many of these rules have since been expanded, the original law applied to businesses with at least 25 employees and labor organizations such as unions. Title VII bans discrimination in firing, hiring, compensation, and other conditions of employment on the grounds of race, color, religion, sex, or national origin. Exceptions include bona fide occupational qualifications and being a member of the Communist Party. Notably, this was the only title to include sex as a protected class after the amendment by Representative Smith. The other titles would be later amended to include sex as a protected class.

Although it was intended to address discrimination in voting registration, Title I did not properly address the barriers to voting faced by Black people and other disenfranchised groups (e.g., poll taxes, literacy tests, violence) and was superseded by the more robust Voting Rights Act of 1965 (VRA). The Twenty-Fourth Amendment, ratified in 1964, put an end to poll taxes. The VRA eliminated other voting qualifications beyond citizenship, including any voting law that would result in discrimination based on race or color. It also required changes in local voting laws in jurisdictions with historically discriminatory voting practices; voting procedures were now subject to federal approval.

More recent pieces of legislation have built on the CRA and expanded civil rights protections. For example, numerous laws aimed to create more equitable and robust educational experiences. Title IX of the Education Amendments Act of 1972 provided protections against discrimination on the basis of sex in programs that receive federal funding. Head Start, a program providing early childhood education and other services for families with young children, was first established in 1965 and was later expanded with federal legislation in the Head Start Act of 1981. Although the CRA started to address educational segregation and the racial achievement gap, it did not speak to residential discrimination. Redlining, the practice by governmental agencies, banks, and other institutions of assigning high risk and low favorability scores to Black and immigrant neighborhoods, was just one of many contributors to housing discrimination in the twentieth century. The Housing and Urban Development Act of 1965 and the Fair Housing Act of 1968 targeted discrimination in housing, and these laws are discussed in Chapter 8, "Remodeling and Breaking New Ground: The Housing and Urban Development Act of 1965."

The Equal Employment Opportunity Act was introduced and enacted in 1972. This legislation offered amendments to Title VII of the CRA. First, it applied the law to smaller employers (those with 15 or more employees) as well as state and local governments, which had been exempt. Second, in response to the backlog of employment discrimination allegations, it restructured and expanded the agency tasked with enforcing the law. Another major amendment to Title VII came with the Civil Rights Act of 1991, signed into law by President George H.W. Bush. Most significantly, proof of intent was no longer a requirement when suing an employer for discriminatory practices. Interestingly, a somewhat more comprehensive bill had been proposed the year before but was vetoed by President Bush, who had been concerned that it would establish hiring quotas in the workplace. The attempt to overturn the veto in the Senate fell short by one vote.

A major change in the landscape of health care delivery came about with the passage of Title XVIII of the Social Security Amendments of 1965, which established Medicare. A federally funded hospital insurance for those older than 65 years, Medicare would serve as a major funding source for hospitals across the country. Even though the separate but equal tenet in the Hill-Burton Act had been overturned in response to *Simkins v. Cone*, the new public insurance program provided a potent means to compel hospital desegregation. The combination of Medicare and Title VI of the CRA meant that hospitals would have to desegregate if they wanted to participate and receive Medicare funding. An army of compliance officers was trained by the Office of Equal Health Opportunity and deployed across the country to assess hospitals' compliance with Title VI. At first, many hospitals in the South resisted, either by refusing to accept Medicare or by trying to find loopholes. This led to a concern that all the seniors who signed up for Medicare in those nonparticipating hospitals' communities would be left without a medical facility. In the end, the national effort by Office of Equal Health Opportunity workers managed to enroll and certify a critical mass of hospitals. By the time Medicare launched on July 1, 1966, 97% of acute-care hospitals were signed on with Medicare (Smith 2016). The few hospitals that were holdouts often experienced financial deterioration while their competitors thrived and expanded.

Many effects of the CRA were not always as rapid as hospital desegregation. Nevertheless, its impacts were far-reaching in many aspects of society, and, as a result, the CRA influenced many social determinants of health and mental health. Many facets of life were affected by the legislation, and those impacts undoubtedly contributed to improved mental health. The CRA established protections for people regardless of race, national origin, religion, and (eventually) sex. It therefore brought forth benefits for many groups that had been historically disadvantaged, including women and people of color. However, given the fact that Black leaders such as Ella Baker took the lead in the civil rights movement—which then drove policy makers to pass the CRA—in the following sections we continue to focus largely on the legislation's impacts on the Black community.

Opening the Door to Better Mental Health

The decades that followed the passage of the CRA were characterized by slow and incomplete waves of racial integration across industries and communities. Compared with many other institutions, schools managed to integrate more. Although *Brown v. Board of Education* laid the groundwork for school desegregation, many school districts did not integrate until they were forced to do so by Title IV and Title VI lawsuits. Ironically, these places of learning tended to avoid any discussion about race; schools around the country did not host assemblies or instruct educators to discuss desegregation. Despite that, interviews of former students from that time reveal that proximity to students of different races greatly reduced their fear and distrust of others (Wells 2004). However, racial divisions persisted in many ways; for example, the most challenging courses were typically available only to white students. Furthermore, integration did not spill into other aspects of everyday life to the same degree. For example, restaurants and many other businesses were required to be open to all people regardless of race, but in the early years, many Black people hesitated to patronize establishments that might potentially be sites of racial conflict (Raskin 2019).

The provisions of the CRA also had economic and occupational implications for the Black community. Before the CRA, if they were lucky enough to be employed, many Black workers had been relegated to physical labor and service jobs such as private cooks and maids in the South. In the North, they were excluded from lucrative industries and cast as inferior workers. After the act's passage, skilled and educated Black people, particularly men, were better able to compete in the job market (Collins 1997). The Black-white wage gap among working men decreased from 50% in 1967 to 30% in 1974 (Couch and Daly 2000), and this contributed to the growth of the Black middle class.

Although the move toward social and economic equity was incomplete and slow, integration did coincide with shifts in racist attitudes among white people in the United States. One key metric of racist attitudes is the explicit desire to maintain distance from and avoid assimilation with stigmatized groups. One longitudinally administered survey asked white respondents if they would have any objection to sending their children to a school where half the students were Black. In 1958, 5 in 10 white parents reported no objection. By 1990, 9 in 10 respondents said they had no issue with that situation (Williams and Williams-Morris 2000). Despite the sentiment expressed in that survey, some white parents today still push back on efforts to integrate schools (Hannah-Jones 2014). Nevertheless, the survey results demonstrate a significant shift in what was acceptable in mainstream white America.

Racism, however, is more than just what white people think or say about Black people. It is better defined as "the system of structuring opportunity and assigning value based on the social interpretation of how one looks (which is what we call 'race'), that unfairly disadvantages some individuals and communities, unfairly advantages other individuals and communities, and saps the strength of the whole society through the waste of human resources" (Jones 2020). Like other systems of oppression, there are multiple levels to racism: systemic, interpersonal, and internalized; each of these affects mental health in different yet connected ways (Jones 2000; Priest and Williams 2018). To the extent that the CRA and related legislation had the effect of addressing different forms of racism and discrimination in the United States, they also affected drivers of mental health.

Systemic Racism

Systemic racism involves discriminatory policies and practices within organizations and on a societal level that result in differential access to goods, services, opportunities, and power. This level encompasses what others have referred to as institutional, structural, and cultural racism (Paradies 2006). At this level, racism affects mental health through a complex interplay of many societal domains. A key example is residential segregation because neighborhood strongly influences educational and occupational opportunities as well as exposures to poverty, violence, trauma, and environmental hazards. Each of these, in turn, has direct impacts on mental health (Figure 6–4).

Longitudinal studies show that improved educational opportunities provided many benefits for Black students. Compared with children who remained in segregated schools, Black students who attended integrated schools achieved better grades and, later in life, better jobs and salaries (Johnson 2011). These outcomes may be further improved when paired with participation in Head Start. In addition, integration did not negatively affect white students' educational attainment. Higher-quality education is associated with enhanced brain development, improved coping mechanisms, and lower rates of depression (Powers 2015). Similarly, the CRA led to a decrease in Black-white income inequality. Declining income inequality is associated with a reduction of depression, self-reported poor mental health, and drug overdose deaths, among other outcomes (Manseau 2015).

The expansion of voting enfranchisement by the VRA potentially affected mental health through direct and indirect means. A direct pathway is the physiological stress response that can occur in reaction to being denied the right to vote, particularly when this is done with violence or the threat of violence (Purtle 2013). Even aside from the potential for violence, the experience of social exclusion can result in stress (Wang et al. 2017). An indirect connection between mental health and voting rights is the inability of a disenfranchised community to advocate for equitable public resources, which, in turn, affects mental health on a community level (Purtle 2013).

Historical practices also affect today's societal landscape and thus are a major contributor to systemic racism. The legacies of some of the most undeniably racist institutions in U.S. history—slavery and the Jim Crow system—had and continue to have direct effects on the mental health of Black Americans. Even though slavery and involuntary servitude were abolished (with the exception of forced labor as part of incarceration after the Civil War), the harms of chattel slavery live on through historical or transgenerational trauma. This has been described as posttraumatic slavery syndrome (DeGruy 2017). Historical trauma can affect the mental health of subsequent generations that did not directly experience the traumatic conditions in multiple ways (Mohatt et al. 2014; Straussner and Calnan 2014), including societal mechanisms, such as the minimizing of narratives of marginalized populations; familial pathways, such as influences on parenting dynamics;

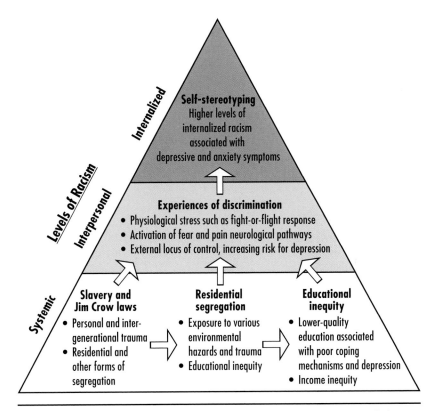

FIGURE 6–4. Examples of the three levels of racism and the ways in which they affect each other and mental health.

The arrows represent some, but not all, of the causal relationships among these types of racism because in actuality, the levels of racism are mutually reinforcing.

and epigenetic changes that can be transmitted intergenerationally. These historical traumas were exacerbated under Jim Crow because Black people had to carefully navigate society in order to avoid confrontation with white people. The pressures of delicately tiptoeing around the racist social norms while risking violence, imprisonment, or worse have been described as segregation stress syndrome (Thompson-Miller et al. 2014). Growing up in this era has been compared with "warlike trauma," but the trauma is more continual, which differentiates segregation stress syndrome from PTSD (Mills and Edwards 2002). Because the CRA prohibited segregation in many settings and helped reduce other overtly racist social norms, it mitigated a major source of continual, intergenerational trauma.

The CRA addressed another aspect of systemic racism: segregated medical care. Desegregating hospitals literally opened the doors for Black patients to obtain more equitable health care. Access to physical health care has been shown to be important for mental health. For example, people who were not able to access general medical care during Superstorm Sandy in the Northeast in 2012 were more likely to have symptoms of depression, anxiety, and PTSD than those who could access care (Ruskin et al. 2018). Furthermore, efforts to desegregate psychiatric hospitals were given more leverage by Title VI, which allowed Black patients to get mental health care at better-funded institutions. Ultimately, the potential benefits of desegregation of psychiatric hospitals were overshadowed by the deinstitutionalization movement (and *transinstitutionalization* into the criminal justice system) that occurred in the years following desegregation (Nuriddin 2019).

Interpersonal Racism

Interpersonal racism, also called personally mediated racism, consists of prejudice and discrimination toward others because of their race (Jones 2000). Studies have found that experiencing racial discrimination has an adverse effect on health in general, with a greater impact on psychological health than physical health (Carter et al. 2017). Psychological sequelae in adults include, but are not limited to, depression, anxiety, and impaired decision-making. Even the anticipation of unfair treatment can lead to an effect as severe as that caused by an observable episode of discrimination (Mays et al. 2007). School-age children and adolescents are also subject to the deleterious mental health effects of experiencing or witnessing racial discrimination. These experiences lead to increased risk of behavioral problems, anxiety, depression, and substance use (Priest and Williams 2018).

Interpersonal racism may affect mental health by many pathways. One is allostatic load, which is a stress response that activates the sympathetic nervous system (i.e., fight-or-flight response), the hypothalamic-pituitary-adrenal axis, and the immune system. Another mechanism arises from repeated experiences of discrimination, which can create an external locus of control, or the perception that outside factors determine one's destiny, leading to a sense of helplessness and reducing adaptive coping responses to stress. Conversely, someone with an internal locus of control perceives that their actions and decisions will determine their future and tends to take positive actions toward managing stress and solving problems. When people have an external rather than an internal locus of control, they are more likely to be depressed and have worse cognition (Zahodne et al. 2015). Last, neuroimaging studies have shown how discrimination alters activation of various regions of the brain. Activity is increased in the amygdala and anterior cingulate cortex, related to fear and pain pathways, respectively, whereas a decrease in prefrontal cortex activity signifies a reduced capacity for executive functioning, planning, and emotional control (Mays et al. 2007).

Internalized Racism

The third level of racism, internalized racism, occurs as individuals in a marginalized group accept societal beliefs about their inferiority (Jones 2000). Multiple studies have demonstrated a correlation between measures of internalized racism and worse mental health. One of these studies (Mouzon and McLean 2017) found that the degree of impact is moderated by at least a few variables. First, high self-esteem and an internal locus of control have a protective effect. Second, Black people born and raised in the Caribbean and living in the United States were affected less than U.S.-born Black people. In other words, growing up in a majority-Black society and being socialized to believe that Black people are not subordinate and can hold positions of power in government is a powerful protective factor. Similarly, researchers have found improved self-perceptions among Black Americans in the context of the election of Barack Obama as the first Black U.S. president (Rivera and Plant 2016). Applied more broadly, this implies that an increase in opportunities for success among the Black community, such as those the CRA provided, is one of many factors that can reduce levels of internalized racism and thus improve mental health.

The effects of racism on mental health are complex, happen on multiple levels, and are moderated by factors that include a sense of empowerment and self-determination. To the extent that the CRA opened up educational and economic opportunities, reduced certain racist attitudes held by white people, and dampened the degree of internalized racism, the law had broad, positive impacts on mental health. It may go without saying that the CRA did not come close to eliminating racism or its effects on mental health, in part because racism has been so entrenched in the nation's institutions and societal fabric and in part because the law was riddled with shortcomings.

"Forty Yards Before the Starting Line"

The main shortcoming of the CRA was that it failed to address inequities that arose from past discrimination. Undoing Jim Crow laws did not magically undo the poverty, discrimination, and other challenges that the Black community faced. Civil rights activists had wanted more from the CRA, specifically policies that would address accumulated advantages that white people had been given, such as in housing, employment, and wealth. When Congress considered one such policy by eliminating the seniority that white workers enjoyed, white labor pushed back. "We don't think that one form of injustice can be corrected or should be corrected by creating another," AFL-CIO lawyer Thomas E. Harris stated in his testimony to Congress. Not addressing seniority and other forms of past inequities was "akin to asking the Negro to enter the 100-yard dash forty yards before the starting line," retorted Carl Rachlin, the general counsel for CORE (Kendi 2017). In the end, that is what the legislators asked of Black people.

Not only was the CRA race blind, but it also failed to recognize the challenges that Black women and other women of color faced. When a recession in the early 1970s led to layoffs, seniority-based policies at companies such as General Motors disadvantaged Black women, who were all hired after the implementation of the CRA. Five Black women sued the company in 1976, but the court ruled against them, stating that Title VII does not recognize Black women as a separate protected class. Kimberlé Crenshaw, who coined the term *intersectionality*, argued that this viewpoint ignores the unique challenges that Black women as a group face (Coaston 2019).

Another shortcoming of the CRA was its lack of policy to curb police brutality, which continued to terrorize Black communities. In response, major protests erupted in the 1960s, most notably in 1965 in Watts, a Black neighborhood in Los Angeles, and in about a dozen more cities the following year. Then, uprisings exploded in more than 100 Black communities across the country in what was dubbed the Long Hot Summer of 1967. In contrast to the nonviolent civil disobedience of SNCC and other organizations, these events led to the deaths of several dozen people and many more injuries. However, in the words of Reverend King, "a riot is the language of the unheard" (Bote 2020). Uprisings are a rational response when communities are continually oppressed and can bring attention and positive policy change to urgent injustices (Lopez 2016).

The death and injury tolls in these events spurred the governor of California at the time, Edmund G. Brown, and President Johnson to order investigations into the causes and solutions of the Watts and 1967 uprisings, respectively. The McCone Commission and Kerner Commission reports that resulted from the investigations both identified similar root causes in the Black community: an unfair judicial system, improper policing practices, substandard housing, high unemployment, and, in general, a racist society (Dawsey 1990; Zelizer 2016). The reports' recommendations to target these underlying issues, which would have essentially addressed social determinants of mental health, were largely not followed by either Governor Brown or President Johnson. Meanwhile, Richard Nixon, who would be Johnson's successor, campaigned on a law-and-order platform, threatening to use force against protestors who did not "respect" the law. Uprisings over ongoing police brutality continue to this day, and mass incarceration, especially of Black men, remains largely unaddressed.

The insufficient action on the part of the government to curb police brutality and to offer solutions to poverty was among the driving forces leading to the emergence of the Black Panther Party (BPP) and the larger

Black Power movement in the mid-1960s. Both groups advocated for Black Americans to shift focus away from integration and instead fight for economic and political self-sufficiency within their community. Although the BPP is remembered for their black berets and militant style, their focus on self-reliance and social mission should not be overlooked. Recognizing that a wide set of services was needed to address the harms perpetuated in oppressed communities, the BPP required its chapters to run "serve the people" programs (i.e., to directly address the social determinants of mental health), including free breakfast programs, free medical clinics, and voter registration drives (Bassett 2016; Choi 2020). Believing that the Black Power movement threatened the status quo of the country, the FBI's counterintelligence program, COINTELPRO, worked to dismantle the movement by infiltrating it, spreading falsehoods about its members, and imprisoning and assassinating its leaders.

While the FBI was covertly disrupting the Black Power movement, President Nixon co-opted the movement's language and rhetoric by launching the "Black capitalism" program. This initiative offered paltry tax credits to incentivize entrepreneurship, a supposed attempt at righting the wrongs perpetrated against the Black community (Coleman 2019). Nixon's top aide would admit decades later that much of the language in Nixon's talking points was, in fact, coded language to appeal to anti-Black voters (Baradaran 2019). Fred Hampton, a BPP leader whose assassination was orchestrated under COINTELPRO, was not fooled by Nixon's rhetoric, stating, "We're gonna fight fire with water. We're gonna fight racism not with racism, but with solidarity. We're not gonna fight capitalism with Black capitalism, but with socialism" (Serrato 2019). Indeed, Nixon's program lacked any meaningful effect when the average Black household in America was struggling to get by, much less start a business. Nevertheless, many presidential administrations that followed (including those of Clinton, Obama, and Trump) used similar approaches, that is, meager tax cuts instead of properly addressing historical and current systemic disadvantage (Baradaran 2019).

Today, we still see the effects of racist policies and practices from before and after the CRA (and the lack of corrective measures). Neighborhoods that were redlined starting in the 1930s remain overwhelmingly Black neighborhoods, and the lack of investment over the past century is still evident. Formerly redlined districts have poorer air quality and worse food access, and because they have fewer trees planted and fewer parks built compared with other districts, they are 5°F–20°F hotter (Plumer et al. 2020). A greater amount of greenery in a neighborhood is correlated with better mental health and social cohesion (Ulmer et al. 2016). The racial wealth gap is another consequence of centuries of racist policies. A great

deal of wealth accumulation comes from home ownership, and Black people have historically been blocked from building wealth because of racist
housing policies. As a result, the median white family is about 10 times
wealthier than the median Black family. In addition, the effects of the CRA
on school desegregation have dwindled over time (Figure 6–5). After federal intervention in the 1970s and 1980s led to peak integration of school
districts in 1988, schools are now by some measures nearly as segregated as
they were before the CRA (Nazaryan 2018), and the racial gap in education,
a major social determinant of mental health, remains a critical problem.

Segregation in health care persists, too, even though the CRA and
Medicare ended legal segregation in hospitals. Black patients are more
likely to be treated at underfunded and overstretched clinics and hospitals.
One study found that nearly half of the Black-white inequity in maternal
mortality in New York City could be explained by the hospitals where
mothers delivered (Howell et al. 2016). Racism in the health care system
manifests in ways other than segregated care. Within the field of psychiatry,
overdiagnosis of schizophrenia among Black people persists to this day as
psychiatrists often diagnose white patients with a less stigmatized mood disorder such as depression or bipolar disorder and Black patients with schizophrenia, even though they exhibit identical symptoms (American Psychiatric
Association 2021; Metzl 2010). In addition, white clinicians may confound
a healthy level of societal mistrust and anger with clinical paranoia and ag-
itation. This seems to be a remnant of psychiatry's historical response to the
civil rights movement, when the diagnostic criteria for schizophrenia were
completely transformed and weaponized against Black people (Metzl
2010). What had previously been a condition describing the docility of predominantly white middle-class housewives was transformed to a disease of
rage supposedly found in Black men.

Protections for voting rights have regressed over the past decade and
have been subject to intense debate recently. After a 2013 Supreme Court
ruling that the part of the VRA of 1965 requiring federal review of changes
to state and local voting laws was no longer enforceable, jurisdictions
around the country have been able to propose and pass without federal
oversight voting restrictions that effectively make it harder for Black citizens to vote (Williams 2021). This is compounded by felony disenfranchisement laws that exist in nearly all states, given that mass incarceration
also has unfairly targeted Black communities for decades. Legislation to restore the VRA was introduced by Representative John Lewis, the late civil
rights activist–turned politician, whose tenure at SNCC was instrumental
in expanding voting rights in the 1960s. After his death in 2020, the new
bill was reintroduced in Congress and named in his honor. On August 24,
2021, the House of Representatives passed the bill by a margin of 219–212,

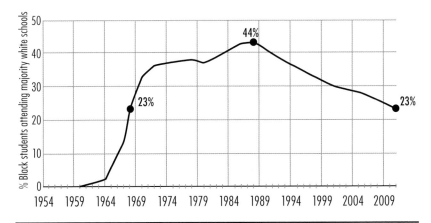

FIGURE 6–5.   School desegregation and resegregation in the South, 1954–2011.

The percentage of Black students in the South attending schools with majority white students reached a peak in 1988. During the 1980s, the Department of Justice under the Reagan and Bush administrations sought to undermine desegregation orders. Furthermore, a 1991 Supreme Court decision weakened the authority of injunctions against school districts. Since then, this marker for school integration has been steadily declining, reaching 23% in 2011, equivalent to the level in 1968. *Source.*   Data from Table 3 of Orfield and Frankenberg 2014.

although, at the time of this writing, it still needs approval by the Senate before it can be signed into law by the president.

The effects of mass incarceration and discriminatory policing are worth a deeper look. After the war on drugs targeted Black communities starting in the 1970s, the federal 1994 Crime Bill coupled with state-level tough-on-crime approaches resulted in a massive explosion in the numbers of incarcerated people, particularly among Black individuals. At the same time, the Clinton administration, aiming to balance the budget, reduced the federal workforce by about 273,000 personnel (Robinson and Wallace 2020). These government positions were held disproportionately by Black people, so the effect of more lost jobs compounded the problem. In addition to losing the right to vote, people with felony records face discrimination in job applications and are ineligible for subsidized housing. The resulting pervasive effects on Black communities—all done under the guise of color-blind polices—have been termed "the new Jim Crow" (Alexander 2010).

More recently, widely shared cell phone camera footage of horrific acts of police brutality and aggressive overpolicing has fueled increasing outrage. Policing in the United States, with its roots in slave patrols and, after the Civil War, enforcement of Jim Crow laws (Hassett-Walker 2021), has continued to harbor racist practices. For instance, Black people are arrested at a rate twice that of white people and are killed by police at six times the rate of white people (Schmidt et al. 2020).

In response to police brutality and other continued patterns of injustice, the Black Lives Matter movement has grown in a way that is reminiscent of Ella Baker's vision for a youth-driven, decentralized movement for justice (Ransby 2015). Its lack of a hierarchical structure does not mean the movement is leaderless but rather, as Black Lives Matter cofounder Patrice Cullors likes to describe it, "leader-full." That is to say, leaders are organizing actions in communities across the country and uplifting local voices that are demanding local and state governments hold police accountable and reduce the overreach of police departments, and, instead, fund social programs in the realms of education, mental health services, and job training. These proposals would target various social determinants of health and mental health. The uprisings across the country in the summer of 2020 have led to some cities passing laws to reform policing and reallocate portions of police agencies' budgets to support social services initiatives (Menjivar 2020).

The CRA paved the way for better protections, resources, and opportunities for many in the Black community and other marginalized populations, but more must be done in pursuit of equality and opportunity for all. After centuries of economic exploitation without an acknowledgment of or remedy for the harms of racial injustice, the calls for truth and reconciliation along with restitution are growing louder. Many different types of policies, falling under the concept of reparations, have been suggested to attempt to level the playing field. One policy proposal, birthright capital, or *baby bonds*, is designed to address the persistent wealth gap. Essentially, the program would set up a trust similar to Social Security, but rather than receiving funds when they retire, Americans would receive up to $60,000 when they turn 18. Because the bulk of the racial wealth gap is derived from disparities in the intergenerational transfer of wealth, the baby trust would reduce the median wealth gap between Black and white young adult households from 16-fold to 1.4-fold (Zewde and Hamilton 2020). As Baker and other civil rights activists pointed out, the CRA did not address poverty, but a birthright capital program could help rectify that shortcoming. Representative John Conyers submitted H.R. 40, a bill that would establish a commission to study various reparation proposals for Black Americans, every year from 1989 until he resigned in 2017. Representative Sheila Jackson Lee has since reintroduced it in 2019 and 2020, and it has gained some momentum (Russ 2019).

In response to the devastating health and economic harms seen during the coronavirus SARS-CoV-2 disease (COVID-19) pandemic, which hit Black communities particularly hard, the American Rescue Plan Act of 2021 had provisions to target poverty and bolster low-income communities. Interestingly, one study's model showed that had a reparations program for Black Americans already been implemented, rates of COVID-19 transmission would have been reduced by 31% to 68% in American communities in general (Andrew 2021). This illustrates one striking example of how reducing or eliminating disparities in wealth would have widespread health benefits. Indeed, a reduction in racial inequality in the United States would improve health, including mental health, for both communities of color and and white communities.

The CRA took aim at some of the most visible and palpable forms of racism and discrimination, clearing the way to a more inclusive society and, in doing so, bringing forth mental health benefits on a societal scale. Yet the road to freedom has been interrupted by detours and setbacks, and racial injustice is still pervasive. Black people are still disproportionately subjected to prison labor (Garcia 2020). Discriminatory law enforcement practices are still reminiscent of the slave patrols from which they originated. Schools are, in fact, becoming *more* segregated. Racial inequities cannot be eliminated without addressing racism, and racism cannot be addressed without acknowledging and rectifying the historical harms that live on today. With hate crimes and other acts of blatant racism becoming more commonplace, making progress in an increasingly polarized nation will be more and more difficult. Nevertheless, understanding past movements for liberation is crucial if we want to move toward a more just, equitable, and healthy society. And civil rights leaders like Ella Baker and John Lewis teach us that progress cannot be made without organizing a sustainable, intergenerational movement that is not afraid to make waves.

References

Alexander M: The New Jim Crow: Mass Incarceration in the Age of Colorblindness. New York, New Press, 2010

American Psychiatric Association: APA's apology to Black, Indigenous, and People of Color for its support of structural racism in psychiatry. Washington, DC, American Psychiatric Association, January 18, 2021. Available at: www.psychiatry.org/newsroom/apa-apology-for-its-support-of-structural-racism-in-psychiatry. Accessed February 10, 2022.

Andrew SC: Reparations for slavery could have reduced Covid-19 transmission and deaths in the US, Harvard study says. Atlanta, GA, CNN, February 16, 2021. Available at: https://edition.cnn.com/2021/02/16/us/reparations-covid-black-americans-disparity-trnd/index.html. Accessed February 10, 2022.

Bagwell O (dir): Eyes on the Prize. Season 1, Episode 3: Ain't Scared of Your Jails: 1960–61. Arlington, VA, PBS, February 4, 1987. Available at: www.pbs.org/video/aint-scared-of-your-jails-1960-1961-sktghc. Accessed February 10, 2022.

Baker EJ: Address at the Hattiesburg Freedom Day rally, in Rhetoric, Religion and the Civil Rights Movement, 1954–1965. Edited by Houck DW, Dixon DE. Amsterdam, Amsterdam University Press, 2006, p 687

Baradaran M: The real roots of "Black capitalism." The New York Times, March 31, 2019. Available at: www.nytimes.com/2019/03/31/opinion/nixon-capitalism-blacks.html. Accessed February 10, 2022.

Bassett MT: Beyond berets: the Black Panthers as health activists. Am J Public Health 106(10):1741–1743, 2016 27626339

Beauchamp Z: The filibuster's racist history, explained. Vox, March 25, 2021. Available at: www.vox.com/policy-and-politics/2021/3/25/22348308. Accessed February 10, 2022.

Bote JUT: "A riot is the language of the unheard": MLK's powerful quote resonates amid George Floyd protests. USA Today, May 29, 2020. Available at: www.usatoday.com/story/news/nation/2020/05/29/minneapolis-protest-martin-luther-king-quote-riot-george-floyd/5282486002. Accessed February 10, 2022.

Carter RT, Lau MY, Johnson V, et al: Racial discrimination and health outcomes among racial/ethnic minorities: a meta-analytic review. J Multicult Couns Devel 45(4):232–259, 2017

Chambers HL: Civil Rights Act of 1964, in Encyclopedia of the Supreme Court of the United States. Edited by Tanenhaus D. New York, Macmillan, 2008, pp 326–331

Choi CH: Educate to liberate: Black Panther liberation schools. New York, The Studio Museum in Harlem, 2020. Available at: https://studiomuseum.org/article/educate-liberate-black-panther-liberation-schools. Accessed January 13, 2021.

Civil Rights Act of 1964, 42 U.S.C. § 2000a et seq.

Coaston J: Intersectionality, explained: meet Kimberlé Crenshaw, who coined the term. Vox, May 28, 2019. Available at: www.vox.com/the-highlight/2019/5/20/18542843/intersectionality-conservatism-law-race-gender-discrimination. Accessed February 10, 2022.

Coleman AR: Black capitalism won't save us. The Nation, May 24, 2019. Available at: www.thenation.com/article/archive/nipsey-killer-mike-race-economics. Accessed February 10, 2022.

Collins SM: Black Corporate Executives. Amsterdam, Amsterdam University Press, 1997

Couch KA, Daly MC: Black-white wage inequality in the 1990s: a decade of progress (Working Paper Series 2000-07). Federal Reserve Bank of San Francisco, August 2000. Available at: www.frbsf.org/economic-research/publications/working-papers/2000/07. Accessed February 10, 2022.

Dawsey D: 25 years after the Watts riots: McCone Commission's recommendations have gone unheeded. Los Angeles Times, July 8, 1990. Available at: www.latimes.com/archives/la-xpm-1990-07-08-me-455-story.html. Accessed March 9, 2019.

DeGruy JA: Post Traumatic Slave Syndrome: America's Legacy of Enduring Injury and Healing. Portland, OR, Joy DeGruy, 2017

Dolen J: Leading from the front. Fort Lauderdale Magazine, February 12, 2020. Available at: https://fortlauderdalemagazine.com/leading-from-the-front. Accessed February 10, 2022.

Education Amendments Act of 1972, 20 U.S.C. § 1681–1688.

Elliott A: Ella Baker: Free agent in the civil rights movement. J Black Stud 26(5):593–603, 1996

Equal Justice Initiative: Reconstruction in America: racial violence after the Civil War, 1865–1876. Montgomery, AL, Equal Justice Initiative, 2020. Available at: https://eji.org/report/reconstruction-in-america. Accessed February 10, 2022.

Garcia T: What does "prison labor" really mean, and should we abolish it? Bustle, June 30, 2020. Available at: www.bustle.com/rule-breakers/what-does-prison-labor-really mean-should-we-abolish-it-27626108. Accessed February 10, 2022.

Grant J (dir): Fundi: The Story of Ella Baker. Brooklyn, NY, Icarus Films, 1981. Available at: https://icarusfilms.com/if-ell2. Accessed February 10, 2022.

Hannah-Jones N: School segregation, the continuing tragedy of Ferguson. New York, ProPublica, December 19, 2014. Available at: www.propublica.org/article/ferguson-school-segregation. Accessed February 9, 2022.

Hassett-Walker C: How you start is how you finish? The slave patrol and Jim Crow origins of policing. Chicago, IL, American Bar Association, January 11, 2021. Available at: www.americanbar.org/groups/crsj/publications/human_rights_magazine_home/civil-rights-reimagining-policing/how-you-start-is-how-you-finish. Accessed February 9, 2022.

Head Start Act of 1981, 42 U.S.C. §105.

Howell EA, Egorova NN, Balbierz A, et al: Site of delivery contribution to Black-white severe maternal morbidity disparity. Am J Obstet Gynecol 215(2):143–152, 2016 27179441

Johnson RC: Long-run impacts of school desegregation and school quality on adult attainments. Cambridge, MA, National Bureau of Economic Research, 2011. Available at: www.nber.org/system/files/working_papers/w16664/w16664.pdf. Accessed February 9, 2022.

Jones CP: Levels of racism: a theoretic framework and a gardener's tale. Am J Public Health 90(8):1212–1215, 2000 10936998

Jones CP: Seeing the water: seven values targets for anti-racism action. Cambridge, MA, Harvard Medical School Center for Primary Care, August 25, 2020. Available at: https://info.primarycare.hms.harvard.edu/blog/seven-values-targets-anti-racism-action. Accessed February 10, 2022.

Kendi IX: The Civil Rights Act was a victory against racism: but racists also won. The Washington Post, July 2, 2017. Available at: www.washingtonpost.com/news/made-by-history/wp/2017/07/02/the-civil-rights-act-was-a-victory-against-racism-but-racists-also-won. Accessed February 10, 2022.

Largent EA: Public health, racism, and the lasting impact of hospital segregation. Public Health Rep 133(6):715–720, 2018 30223719

Lopez G: Riots are destructive, dangerous, and scary—but can lead to serious social reforms. Vox, September 22, 2016. Available at: www.vox.com/2015/4/30/8518681/protests-riots-work. Accessed February 10, 2022.

Manseau MW: Economic inequality, poverty, and neighborhood deprivation, in The Social Determinants of Mental Health. Edited by Compton MT, Shim RS. Arlington, VA, American Psychiatric Association Publishing, 2015, pp 121–144

Mays VM, Cochran SD, Barnes NW: Race, race-based discrimination, and health outcomes among African Americans. Annu Rev Psychol 58(1):201–225, 2007 16953796

McGreevy N: Five things to know about the 1876 presidential election. Smithsonian Magazine, January 5, 2021. Available at: www.smithsonianmag.com/smart-news/confusion-voter-suppression-and-constitutional-crisis-five-things-know-about-1876-presidential-election-180976677. Accessed February 14, 2022.

Menjivar J: Black Lives Matter protests: what's been achieved so far. New York, Do-Something.org, August 13, 2020. Available at: www.dosomething.org/us/articles/black-lives-matter-protests-whats-been-achieved-so-far. Accessed February 14, 2022.

Metzl JM: The Protest Psychosis. Amsterdam, Amsterdam University Press, 2010

Mills TL, Edwards CDA: A critical review of research on the mental health status of older African-Americans. Ageing Soc 22(3):273–304, 2002

Mohatt NV, Thompson AB, Thai ND, et al: Historical trauma as public narrative: a conceptual review of how history impacts present-day health. Soc Sci Med 106:128–136, 2014 24561774

Mouzon DM, McLean JS: Internalized racism and mental health among African-Americans, US-born Caribbean Blacks, and foreign-born Caribbean Blacks. Ethn Health 22(1):36–48, 2017 27354264

Nazaryan A: School segregation in America is as bad today as it was in the 1960s. Newsweek, March 23, 2018. Available at: www.newsweek.com/2018/03/30/school-segregation-america-today-bad-1960–855256.html. Accessed February 14, 2022.

Nuriddin A: Psychiatric Jim Crow: desegregation at the Crownsville State Hospital, 1948–1970. J Hist Med Allied Sci 74(1):85–106, 2019 30476136

O'Donnell M: How LBJ saved the Civil Rights Act. The Atlantic, April 2014. Available at: www.theatlantic.com/magazine/archive/2014/04/what-the-hells-the-presidency-for/358630. Accessed February 14, 2022.

Onion R: The real story behind "because of sex." Slate Magazine, June 16, 2020. Available at: slate.com/news-and-politics/2020/06/title-vii-because-of-sex-howard-smith-history.html. Accessed February 14, 2022.

Orfield G, Frankenberg E: Brown at 60: great progress, a long retreat and an uncertain future. Los Angeles, CA, Civil Rights Project/Proyecto Derechos Civiles, May 15, 2014. Available at: https://civilrightsproject.ucla.edu/research/k-12-education/integration-and-diversity/brown-at-60-great-progress-a-long-retreat-and-an-uncertain-future/Brown-at-60-051814.pdf. Accessed February 14, 2022.

Paradies YC: Defining, conceptualizing and characterizing racism in health research. Crit Public Health 16(2):143–157, 2006

Plessy v Ferguson, 163 US 537 (1896)

Plumer B, Popovich N, Palmer B: How decades of racist housing policy left neighborhoods sweltering. The New York Times, August 24, 2020. Available at: www.nytimes.com/interactive/2020/08/24/climate/racism-redlining-cities-global-warming.html. Accessed February 14, 2022.

Powers RA: Poor education, in The Social Determinants of Mental Health. Edited by Compton MT, Shim RS. Arlington, VA, American Psychiatric Association Publishing, 2015, pp 77–98

Priest N, Williams DR: Racial discrimination and racial disparities in health, in The Oxford Handbook of Stigma, Discrimination, and Health. Edited by Major B, Dovidio JF, Link BG. New York, Oxford University Press, 2018, pp 163–182

Purtle J: Felon disenfranchisement in the United States: a health equity perspective. Am J Public Health 103(4):632–637, 2013 23153146

Ransby B: Ella Baker and the Black Freedom Movement: A Radical Democratic Vision. Chapel Hill, University of North Carolina Press, 2003

Ransby B: Ella Baker's radical democratic vision. Jacobin, June 18, 2015. Available at: www.jacobinmag.com/2015/06/black-lives-matter-police-brutality. Accessed February 14, 2022.

Raskin H: Charleston-area residents remember the first time they ate in white-owned restaurants. The Post and Courier, May 18, 2019. Available at: www.postandcourier.com/article_608fe684-3570-11e9-9169-77939a8 e4144.html. Accessed February 14, 2022.

Rivera LM, Plant EA: The psychological legacy of Barack Obama: the impact of the first African-American president of the United States on individuals' social cognition. Soc Cogn 34(6):495–503, 2016

Robinson J, Wallace C: The myth of post-racial America, in Who We Are: A Chronicle of Racism in America, Episode 6 (podcast). Vox Creative, October 20, 2020. Available at: www.vox.com/ad/21354746/who-we-are-podcast-racism-in-america. Accessed February 14, 2022.

Ruskin J, Rasul R, Schneider S, et al: Lack of access to medical care during Hurricane Sandy and mental health symptoms. Prev Med Rep 10:363–369, 2018 29868393

Russ V: What you need to know about reparations after the first congressional hearing convened on the topic in more than a decade. The Philadelphia Inquirer, June 22, 2019. Available at: www.inquirer.com/news/what-are-reparations-america-h-r-40-congressional-hearings-democratic-presidential-candidates-20190619.html. Accessed February 14, 2022.

Schmidt L, Haskell-Hoehl M, McGill K, et al: Data-backed outrage: police violence by the numbers. Vera Institute of Justice, July 7, 2020. Available at: www.vera.org/blog/target-2020/data-backed-outrage-police-violence-by-the-numbers. Accessed August 26, 2020.

Serrato J: Fifty years of Fred Hampton's Rainbow Coalition. South Side Weekly, September 27, 2019. Available at: https://southsideweekly.com/fifty-years-fred-hampton-rainbow-coalition-young-lords-black-panthers. Accessed February 14, 2022.

Smith DB: The Power to Heal: Civil rights, Medicare, and the Struggle to Transform America's Health Care System. Nashville, TN, Vanderbilt University Press, 2016

Straussner SL, Calnan AJ: Trauma through the life cycle: a review of current literature. Clin Soc Work J 42(4):323–335, 2014

Thompson-Miller R, Feagin JR, Picca LH: Jim Crow's Legacy: The Lasting Impact of Segregation (Perspectives on a Multiracial America). New York, Rowman & Littlefield, 2014

Ulmer JM, Wolf KL, Backman DR, et al: Multiple health benefits of urban tree canopy: the mounting evidence for a green prescription. Health Place 42:54–62, 2016 27639106

Voting Rights Act of 1965, 52 U.S.C. § 10101.

Wang H, Braun C, Enck P: How the brain reacts to social stress (exclusion)—a scoping review. Neurosci Biobehav Rev 80:80–88, 2017 28535967

Wells AS: How desegregation changed us: the effects of racially mixed schools on students and society. New York, Teachers College, Columbia University, October14, 2004. Available at: www.tc.columbia.edu/articles/2004/march/how-desegregation-changed-us-the-effects-of-racially-mixed-. Accessed February 9, 2022.

Williams DR, Williams-Morris R: Racism and mental health: the African American experience. Ethn Health 5(3–4):243–268, 2000 11105267

Williams R: John Lewis Voting Rights Act could thwart state plans to curb access. Georgia Recorder, January 25, 2021. Available at: https://georgiarecorder.com/2021/01/25/john-lewis-voting-rights-act-could-thwart-state-plans-to-curb-access. Accessed February 14, 2022.

Zahodne LB, Meyer OL, Choi E, et al: External locus of control contributes to racial disparities in memory and reasoning training gains in ACTIVE. Psychol Aging 30(3):561–572, 2015 26237116

Zelizer JE: Is America repeating the mistakes of 1968 and ignoring structural racism? The Atlantic, July 9, 2016. Available at: www.theatlantic.com/politics/archive/2016/07/is-america-repeating-the-mistakes-of-1968/490568. Accessed February 14, 2022.

Zewde N, Hamilton D: Truth and redistribution. YES! Magazine, August 26, 2020. Available at: www.yesmagazine.org/issue/black-lives/2020/08/26/racial-wealth-gap-black-power. Accessed February 14, 2022.

Zinn H: SNCC: The New Abolitionists, 2nd Edition. Boston, MA, Beacon Press, 1965

7 | The Times They Are A-Changin'

The Elementary and Secondary Education Act of 1965

Rebecca A. Powers, M.D., M.P.H.

Two Different Browns: The Beginnings of a Fight

Esther Brown was a 30-year-old Jewish housewife in Merriam, Kansas. She was upset that an all-Black school in the South Park neighborhood of her African American maid was in dreadful condition. The students at the 88-year-old two-room Walker School had to use an outhouse on the dirt playground, walk home for lunch, and attend a school with no principal and only two teachers. In 1948, she began a fight for racial justice in this Kansas school district (Katz and Tucker 1995). Mrs. Brown took complaints to an all-white school board that was currently trying to create a new school for white students. They were so disinterested that they settled on giving the school for Black students two new light bulbs, and Mrs. Brown left the meeting enraged by their absurd concession (Linder 2011). This was the state of educational inequality in America in 1948.

165

Mrs. Brown continued her pursuit, not necessarily for integration, but just for a fair shake. She led meetings for African American parents and asked that white parents also join her cause. She asked the Kansas City chapter of the National Association for the Advancement of Colored People (NAACP) to file suit and then raised money for the legal battle. She got the word out everywhere she could—even at a Billie Holliday concert. She was not happy with her first counsel, so she fired him and hired Black Topeka attorney Elisha Scott to take on the case against the South Park district. A trailblazer, she pushed for a boycott of the all-Black school and set up worthy new private schools to educate the Black students instead (Linder 2011). Her activism cost her, however. A cross was burned in her yard, her husband was fired from his job, and she had several threats against her life. This was the state of American society in the late 1940s. Mrs. Brown was persistent nonetheless, and her cause prevailed. In 1949, in *Webb v. School District No. 90*, the Kansas Supreme Court determined that Black students had the right to attend a new, previously all-white South Park school. This decision would be the prelude to an even more impactful court ruling.

Now meet another Brown. Oliver Brown, a resident of Topeka, Kansas, was an assistant pastor at St. Mark's African Methodist Episcopal Church and a welder for the railroad (National Park Services 2021). In 1952, when he was in his early 30s, he and his wife had three children, ages 8 years, 4 years, and 5 months. His daughter, Linda, attended the all-Black Monroe Elementary School located 21 blocks from their home. Mr. Brown testified that "many times [Linda] had to wait through cold, the rain, and the snow" for a bus to take her to Monroe. There was an all-white elementary school only 7 blocks away from where they lived. The white students could easily walk to their nearby school. One year prior, the public school district refused to enroll Linda in the school closest to their home.

In 1952, in *Brown v. Board of Education of Topeka*, arguments were brought before the U.S. Supreme Court against the city's Board of Education. It was argued that Mr. Brown's daughter's school was not the same as others in the district but rather was inherently unequal. Americans watched as the court prepared to tackle the almost six-decade-old doctrine of "separate but equal" segregation. Across the country, the movement to desegregate public institutions was gaining traction.

Although the suit had multiple plaintiffs, Oliver Brown's name preceded the others alphabetically; as such, his name is forever attached to it (Figure 7–1). Brown became the outward face of the lawsuit to the media. When it was finally decided in 1954, *Brown v. Board of Education of Topeka* became a landmark case in American history. In the District Court of Kansas, judges had previously ruled 3–0 against Brown because the schools were deemed separate but equal. The NAACP lawyers representing the Browns then appealed all the way to the U.S. Supreme Court, and there, they won. The court ruled, unanimously, that U.S. laws establishing segregation in public schools were unconstitutional. This held true, moreover, even if the segregated schools' teaching and physical facilities were equal in quality. "Separate educational facilities," wrote Chief Justice Earl Warren, were "inherently unequal" and thus violated the Equal Protection Clause of the Fourteenth Amendment of the U.S. Constitution (Figure 7–2). The de jure integration that followed was a major victory for the civil rights movement.

By the time the Supreme Court announced its decision pertaining to the desegregation of schools, Linda had moved on to an already integrated junior high school. Fortunately, with the court's new doctrine, her younger siblings could enjoy the benefits of a desegregated elementary education. The outward face of the lawsuit stuck, and since then, the Brown name has become a byword for the desegregation campaign. In 1959, Oliver Brown and his family moved to Springfield, Missouri, where he served as a minister. He died in Springfield of a heart attack in 1961.

Education and Educational Inequality in the Years After the Two Browns

"Noisy and stubborn" came the reaction to the court's ruling in the Deep South, where racial segregation remained deeply entrenched. This "Massive Resistance," led in Congress by Virginia Senator Harry Byrd, intended to frustrate attempts to desegregate Southern schools (Virginia Museum of History and Culture 2021). In 1957, at the height of Massive Resistance, the integration of Central High School in Little Rock, Arkansas, had to be enforced by federal troops. The local resistance to desegregation gained national attention when Governor Orval Faubus sent in the Arkansas National Guard, against court order, to prevent nine African American students from gaining lawful entry into the school. President Dwight D. Eisenhower tried to negotiate with Faubus several times but finally had to take action against the defiant governor, ordering a thousand troops from the U.S. Army in Kentucky to oversee the integration against Faubus's state guard. The Little Rock Nine, as the public dubbed them, entered the academically renowned high school, which hosted an enrollment of about 2,000 white students (Jayne 2020). These brave young people went through torment and discrimination from their classmates, but by the end of the year, eight of the nine remained at Central High School.

Throughout the 1960s and 1970s, integration continued, albeit not always smoothly. Housing patterns brought about by property value disparities, redlining of neighborhoods, and restricting of resources to Black families, as well as other persistent inequities, meant that many cities re-

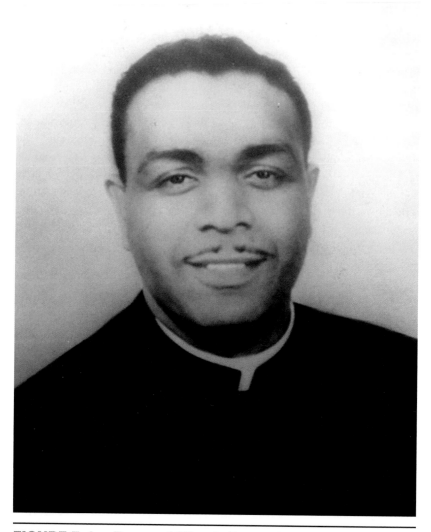

FIGURE 7–1.   Reverend Oliver L. Brown, lead plaintiff in the *Brown v. Board of Education* case.

Source.   National Park Service: Rev. Oliver L. Brown. Available at: www.nps.gov/people/oliver-brown.htm. Accessed July 18, 2022.

mained segregated, which made many school districts de facto segregated. In response, authorities in some states and cities developed programs of forced busing for school children. Many white parents resisted, preferring to have their kids educated in their own neighborhood schools, especially in northern cities. Although theoretical equality in education had been achieved by 1970, full equality and parity in education has still not been fully realized. Integra-

1, 2, 4 & 10

BROWN *v.* BOARD OF EDUCATION.   11

guage in *Plessy* v. *Ferguson* contrary to this finding is rejected.

We conclude that in the field of public education the doctrine of "separate but equal" has no place. Separate educational facilities are inherently unequal. Therefore, we hold that the plaintiffs and others similarly situated for whom the actions have been brought are, by reason of the segregation complained of, deprived of the equal protection of the laws guaranteed by the Fourteenth Amendment. This disposition makes unnecessary any discussion whether such segregation also violates the Due Process Clause of the Fourteenth Amendment.[12]

Because these are class actions, because of the wide applicability of this decision, and because of the great variety of local conditions, the formulation of decrees in these cases presents problems of considerable complexity. On reargument, the consideration of appropriate relief was necessarily subordinated to the primary question— the constitutionality of segregation in public education. We have now announced that such segregation is a denial of the equal protection of the laws. In order that we may have the full assistance of the parties in formulating decrees, the cases will be restored to the docket, and the parties are requested to present further argument on Questions 4 and 5 previously propounded by the Court for the reargument this Term.[13]   The Attorney General

---

[12] See *Bolling* v. *Sharpe, infra,* concerning the Due Process Clause of the Fifth Amendment.

[13] "4. Assuming it is decided that segregation in public schools violates the Fourteenth Amendment

"(*a*) would a decree necessarily follow providing that, within the limits set by normal geographic school districting, Negro children should forthwith be admitted to schools of their choice, or

"(*b*) may this Court, in the exercise of its equity powers, permit an effective gradual adjustment to be brought about from existing segregated systems to a system not based on color distinctions?

"5. On the assumption on which questions 4 (*a*) and (*b*) are

---

FIGURE 7–2.   **Excerpt from the Supreme Court ruling in *Brown v. Board of Education.***

Source.   National Archives: Opinion, 5/17/1954, Case File for *Brown et al. v. Board of Education of Topeka et al.*, Appellate Jurisdiction Case Files, 1792–2017, Record Group 267: Records of the Supreme Court of the United States, 1772–2007. https://catalog.archives.gov/id/1656510, accessed June 20, 2022.

tion efforts began to wane in that decade, reached their final peak in the 1980s, and have gradually declined ever since, although some school districts are still under integration mandates of local courts to this day.

Schools are important for everyone. They serve two main constituencies: students, teaching them how to excel in life, and, more broadly, the community as a whole, cultivating civic values for all and preparing citizens to be productive members of society, regardless of age, race, or other demographics. This dual function matters, especially when considering the most rural and the most urban schools. In most geographic areas, schools are the largest employer; they also claim the largest share of local taxes. They are often the only places that hold community events and are open to the public. Even though schools hold high social importance, educational attainment by Americans in the mid-twentieth century was the exception rather than the rule. The U.S. Department of Agriculture's Economic Research Service determined that in 1960, well over half of students never finished high school. In that year, almost 57% of urban students did not receive a high school diploma; by 2000, however, that number had dropped to 18.8%, and by 2019, it dropped further to 11.7% (U.S. Department of Agriculture 2021). Looking at rural areas, the numbers look even worse. In 1960, more than 66% of rural students nationwide did not graduate high school; in 2000 that number had dropped to 23.7%, and by 2019 it was 13.6% (U.S. Department of Agriculture 2021).

Rural schools in the 1950s and 1960s faced a different type of pressure than those in major cities. When the Soviet satellite Sputnik first orbited the Earth, both an arms race and an educational race began. Newspaper headlines stressed that the United States did not have enough missiles to defend itself—or enough engineers to build the missiles needed. American policy placed math and science at the forefront of schools' educational programs in order to catch up with the Soviet Union. However, many people had been leaving rural areas and moving to urban areas in search of economic opportunity, leaving the potential pool of qualified teachers shallow. Therefore, rural schools were generally smaller and had only a few teachers, who were often not skilled enough to teach math and science well or who were required to teach multiple subjects. In the 1950s, rural educational policy reflected the idea that in order to get the best-qualified teachers, small schools would need to be consolidated. The number of school districts went from 128,000 in 1930 to only 16,000 in 1977 (Ganzel 2007). Teachers, equipment, and administrators were now pooled, and teachers and administrators were more easily professionalized. Districts also started to share resources, allowing for the hiring of specialty teachers in music, art, foreign languages, and physical and special education. These teachers traveled to different districts on different days to provide these specialized classes to all the schools in a region. Of course, these changes met resistance because some rural communities were so isolated that young children would have to ride for hours on the bus to get to and from school.

Then, thinking changed, and educational theorists realized that small schools might well support a better system of education than larger ones by having a lower student-to-teacher ratio and thus giving students more personalized instruction. Indeed, for instance, during the 1960s, studies showed that students in smaller schools were 3–20 times more likely to participate in extracurricular activities than were those at larger schools in urban areas (Holland and Andre 1987). More activities were available in the larger urban schools, but fewer students were able to take advantage of them proportionally. Students from smaller schools fared better on standardized tests, it seemed, especially in the core disciplines, whereas students from urban schools did better when assessed for specialized knowledge.

Aside from rural and urban differences, in the mid-1960s, President Lyndon B. Johnson's Great Society programs related to education broke schools into "disadvantaged" versus "nondisadvantaged" categories. This change in the federal government's education program cut across all urban and rural divides. Now what mattered to the policy's classification of schools, whether urban or rural, was the number of poor students served. Later, further legislation would establish programs for special populations, such as migrant students (e.g., the Migrant Education Program, which was a 1966 amendment to Title I of the 1965 Elementary and Secondary Education Act) and students with disabilities (e.g., the Education for All Handicapped Children Act in 1975, which was later renamed during a reauthorization as the Individuals with Disabilities Education Act).

War on Poverty and the Great Society: A Renewed Movement Toward Equality

The federal law that will be highlighted here, the Elementary and Secondary Education Act of 1965, cannot be understood without an appreciation of the 1960s societal and political context from which it was born. Bob Dylan's 1964 hit song "The Times They Are a-Changin'" could be the tagline for the 1960s. Dylan wrote the song as an attempt to depict and influence people's views of the decade, and, indeed, the decade following *Brown v. Board of Education* brought great social, political, and economic change to the United States. The seeds of activism planted by Esther Brown, Oliver Brown, and other committed activists began well before the 1960s, and over that decade, they continued, flowered, and bore fruit. Throughout the 1960s, a succession of social movements sought to stamp out inequalities in America. The civil rights movement, the women's movement, the counterculture movements, and the Stonewall Rebellion would all change the face of the nation forever.

In 1964, President Lyndon B. Johnson (Figure 7–3) declared the start to a War on Poverty—not a short or easy battle, but a necessary one to ame-

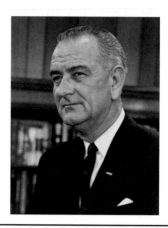

FIGURE 7–3.   President Lyndon B. Johnson.
Source. National Archives. Available at www.archives.gov/research/census/
presidents/lb-johnson.html. Accessed June 21, 2022. Public domain.

liorate current as well as future poverty in a rich nation. Johnson planned
to establish several federal programs to improve everything from health
care to education to job training in America. The War on Poverty was part
of Johnson's bigger vision for the nation, which he called the Great Society.
This Great Society could not discriminate, and by extension, poverty could
not exist. Over the course of just a few years in the mid-1960s, Johnson and
Congress constructed and waged a great legislative campaign, seeking to
obtain this improved, if not ideal, society.

President Johnson introduced the War on Poverty during his State of the
Union address in 1964. He proposed a set of legislation in response to the national poverty rate, which approached a staggering 19% at the time. He argued
that this degree of poverty was a national disgrace for a country with such great
means and that the primary cause could not be construed as a personal failing
of the poor but was rather due to a pervasive, deeply rooted societal failure. To
obtain the Great Society, Johnson believed that the federal government should
play a greater role in education and health care in order to reduce national poverty. "Our aim is not only to relieve the symptom of poverty," Johnson said as
he addressed the nation, "but to cure it and, above all, to prevent it."

The War on Poverty began not only as the personal project of President
Johnson but also as an outcome of the growing recognition of the poverty
problem as detailed in publications in the early 1960s. Poverty was more
prevalent than many people had commonly assumed, and vigorous public
debate of various policy solutions ensued. The civil rights movement in
particular deserves most of the credit for spurring action to address poverty.

The collection of data on national poverty, surprisingly, started only in 1959, as the movement's public pressure increased. The War on Poverty began at a time when escalating involvement in the Vietnam War consumed much of the nation's attention, as well as its economic, social, and political resources; both wars brought about intense deliberation within society. Polarization over issues of national policy developed, and social movements formed to attempt to abolish inequalities in all areas of life. It was out of this turbulent milieu that the civil rights movement emerged.

The movement's goals were much broader than addressing only poverty, and its achievements touched all reaches of American policy deeply. Starting decades before, the movement had aimed to enforce constitutional and legal rights for African Americans that white Americans already enjoyed. Supporters obtained their largest legislative gains in the mid-1960s, during the Johnson presidency. Grassroots protests dating from the mid-1950s led to organized social movements and strategies to end Jim Crow laws dictating racial segregation, disenfranchisement, and discrimination across the United States. Dialogue arose between activists and government authorities after many repeated acts of nonviolent protest, direct action, and civil disobedience. As tensions mounted, the persisting inequities faced by African Americans across the country became a dominant issue of the time. The resulting federal laws aimed to protect all Americans from discrimination on several different fronts, such as education, employment, and housing.

Beyond the War on Poverty and the civil rights movement, several other cultural movements set the context for educational reform—and the Elementary and Secondary Education Act of 1965—in the United States. The women's movement confronted pay disparity in the workplace and argued for more opportunities for women to contribute to the nation's social, economic, and political life. Second-wave feminism, as the reformed movement was called, began in the early 1960s and expanded greatly on the first wave, which had focused on suffrage and equal property rights decades prior. With the renewed second wave, feminists tackled such issues as sexuality, family, the workplace, reproductive rights, and official legal inequalities. This movement also targeted social ills such as domestic violence and marital rape, helping to create resources such as women's shelters and rape crisis centers. In 1960, the FDA approved the combined oral contraceptive pill, allowing many women to continue careers without having to leave work because of an unplanned pregnancy. In 1973, the *Roe v. Wade* Supreme Court decision made abortion legal through the country (until it was reversed by the Supreme Court in June 2022). Women's health, women's employment, women's studies, and childcare all came to the public forefront in ways the nation had never before witnessed.

The countercultural movement also became widespread across the country in the 1960s. New styles of television, cinema, and radio programming all became means by which society could learn and be reshaped, and through them a new popular culture began to form, with new music, new tastes, and new social norms. Opposition coalesced against the Vietnam War. Young people burned their draft cards or moved to Canada. Social tensions developed around many issues, including gender roles, traditional modes of authority, and experimentation with psychoactive drugs. The plight of the poor and the destruction of the environment were in the spotlight. A more tolerant and inclusive social landscape was being forged. The Stonewall Rebellion in New York City in 1969, along with other protests around the same time across the country, sparked awareness of the need for equal rights for lesbian, gay, bisexual, and transgender Americans, who had not seen equality upheld by the rule of law. The broad educational reform of the 1960s, then, did not occur in isolation.

In addition to these cultural changes in society (social norms), major advances were taking place in federal legislation (public policies), many of which directly or indirectly targeted the nation's public systems pertaining to voting, housing, health care, and the like. The Civil Rights Act of 1964 banned discrimination in many facets of life based on color, race, religion, sex, or national origin. This act and subsequent civil rights legislation also ended unequal application of voter registration requirements. Following through on *Brown v. Board of Education*, the act also prohibited racial segregation in schools, the workplace, and public accommodations. Other civil rights gains included the Voting Rights Act of 1965, which restored and protected voting rights for people of color, and the Fair Housing Act of 1968, which banned discrimination in the sale or rental of housing. The Fair Housing Act in particular aimed to address the de facto segregation that persisted across the country, itself a continuing cause of educational segregation and inequality.

The Social Security Amendments of 1965 established Medicare and Medicaid. They expanded Social Security benefits for retirees, widows, persons with disabilities, and college-age young adults. Shortly before, the Food Stamp Act of 1964 had made the then temporary food stamps program permanent, and the program ultimately evolved into today's Supplemental Nutrition Assistance Program (SNAP). The Economic Opportunity Act, also in 1964, established the Job Corps, the Volunteers in Service to America (VISTA) program (a domestic counterpart to the Peace Corps), the federal work-study program, and other employment opportunities for Americans. It also created the federal preschool system, Head Start.

The Office of Economic Opportunity (OEO), established in 1964, was instrumental in overseeing most of the Johnson administration's funds for these programs. Several of these programs persist to this day as continued federal initiatives sparked by the War on Poverty, such as Head Start, VISTA, TRIO, the Legal Services Program, the Community Action Program, and Job Corps, to name a few of the most important. TRIO—initially the combination of Upward Bound, Talent Search, and Student Support Services—was the first set of national college access and retention initiatives to address the serious social and cultural barriers to higher education in America.

The OEO's programs spanned from preschool to postgraduation. It began Project Head Start in 1965. That initiative introduced preschool-age children from low-income families to a program that could meet emotional, social, health, nutritional, and psychological needs. In 1967, the Johnson administration introduced Project Follow Through, which would become the largest educational experiment ever conducted. As befits its name, the study followed up on children enrolled in the Head Start program for years after it began.

The OEO's Job Corps began in 1964 as a program to train disadvantaged and at-risk youth. It integrated academic, vocational, and social skills to offer them independence, a good education, and well-paying long-term jobs. The Job Corps trained youth in conservation camps and urban centers. The U.S. government still offers Job Corps vocational training, as well as high school equivalency programs, high school diplomas, and other means to help disadvantaged students enter college. With Head Start and Job Corps as two bookends, we now highlight the major policy development for the elementary, middle, and high school years.

Elementary and Secondary Education Act of 1965

The nation's campaign against poverty would need to target education in the form of a momentous promise: equal access to quality education, regardless of socioeconomic status and other factors such as English language and disability status. With the Elementary and Secondary Education Act of 1965 (ESEA), this campaign neared realization. This statute funded primary and secondary education, and it emphasized high standards and accountability. It authorized funds for professional development, instructional materials, resources to support educational programs, and the promotion of parental involvement. It sought to shrink achievement gaps between students because each child would receive fair and equal opportunities for exceptional education. From 1965 to 1980, the act was reauthorized every 3 years, with an emphasis on how funds were to be allocated. In total, it has been reauthorized eight times to date. For example, in 2001, the reauthorization of the

1965 act by President George W. Bush was known as the No Child Left Behind Act (NCLB; Klein 2015), and President Barack Obama renewed the bill in 2015 as the Every Student Succeeds Act (U.S. Department of Education 2022). Across the decades, many revisions and amendments have been introduced. The ESEA became the most extensive act affecting education that Congress ever passed.

The ESEA, one of the cornerstones of the Great Society, would address the achievement gaps between disadvantaged students and advantaged ones, one of the most significant inequalities of American society. The ESEA was central to the War on Poverty because, as the Johnson administration knew, improved educational opportunities for all children could help to decrease and prevent poverty in America. Local schools would now receive increased federal funds and involvement, although local districts would retain much flexibility in the use of these funds, which would first be distributed to the states as grants. Several titles were included in this landmark act of Congress, and they are briefly summarized here.

Title I of the ESEA provides for the distribution of funds to schools and school districts with a high percentage of low-income families. Five-sixths of the funding for the ESEA was authorized for Title I. Funds are first allocated by the federal Department of Education to state educational agencies, which then distribute them to local educational agencies, which in turn fund the public schools with the greatest need. The provision also benefits children from families that have immigrated to the United States, as well as youth from intervention programs who have been neglected or abused or who are at risk of abuse. This important title also addresses the prevention of dropping out and the improvement of schools. Eligibility for Title I funding requires that at least 40% of a school's student body come from families with low income. Schools receive priority if they can show obvious need in terms of money, records of low achievement, and commitments to improve their standards and test scores.

Title I provides assistance through two types of programs within the schools that qualify: the *schoolwide program* allows resource use in a flexible manner to implement reforms to upgrade the entire educational program of the school, and the *targeted assistance program* requires schools to direct funds to those students who are failing or most at risk of failing (U.S. Department of Education 2016). Funding is based on the school's specific commitments to improve their system, and schools must submit an application to request these funds. The Title I funding approach—aligned with other efforts to address poverty—was justified because studies have shown an inverse relationship between student achievement and the extent of poverty among a school's students. That is, the expected association between income and educational achievement holds true not only at the individual level but also at the overall school (student body) level.

Over the years, Title I assistance has helped several million children. Most funds, about 60%, are spent on kindergarten through fifth-grade students, and the next highest amount is spent on those in the sixth through eighth grades. High schoolers received the next highest amount of funding, and preschoolers received the least—at about 3%. Even though Title I still exists, the federal government has changed its terms greatly over the six decades since its inception. For the first 15 years of the ESEA, it was reauthorized every 3 years, and its funds were reallocated on the basis of strict federal eligibility rules. If schools were found to be out of compliance, they received punitive action. The government intended Title I funds as ancillary resources and not as replacements for local funds. If 40% or more of a student body was made up of low-income students, then the whole school could receive assistance (the schoolwide program), rather than the targeted approach for specific populations of students with the most need.

The Reagan administration and Congress passed the Education Consolidation and Improvement Act in 1981 to reduce federal funding to Title I. They felt that state and local jurisdictions, rather than the federal government, should provide and control education resources. Even though this law passed, the traditional Title I practices of funding distribution described above continued. Then, in the late 1980s, achievement became the main focus of federal education policy. With new updates to the legislation, the achievement standards for low-income students were raised; advanced skills, compared with basic reading, writing, and mathematics, grew more important, and schools came to expect increased parental involvement in their students' education. If students failed to improve, educators were expected to institute modifications in their approaches as well as to implement broader, schoolwide projects.

In 1994, under President Bill Clinton, the Improving America's Schools Act (IASA) came about to address unsuccessful alterations to Title I in the 1980s. With the IASA, the federal government once again revisited Title I of the ESEA. This amendment would prove to be the last major alteration before the George W. Bush administration's complete overhaul of the law, 2001's NCLB. Clinton's IASA attempted to improve instruction for all students and, moreover, coordinate federal, state, and local funding to do so. Three major changes were made to the ESEA in the IASA of 1994. First, schools would now measure accountability by adding math and reading/language arts standards. Second, by the 1996–1997 school year, only 50% of students had to be low income for a school to use Title I funds on a schoolwide basis, down from previous standards of 75% and 60% in earlier years.

Third, the IASA offered more local control so that federal requirements would not interfere as much with the minutiae of school improvements.

NCLB, another major alteration to the ESEA, came in 2001, during the George W. Bush administration. NCLB increased requirements of accountability from the schools receiving ESEA funding, from their teachers, and from their students. The NCLB mandated yearly standardized tests, expected annual reports showing achievement and sociodemographic changes, and called for corrective actions if investigation determined any misuse of funds at participating schools. The law also required restructuring if schools did not perform adequately; additionally, teachers had to be highly qualified if the school hired them using Title I funds. NCLB, Part A, also allowed private schools to receive Title I funds if they were eligible.

Today, Title I funds can help to purchase electronic devices, to ensure that low-income families have internet access at home, to provide remediation or other informational instruction over the internet at home if needed, and to offer other educational technologies necessary to keep low-income children's education competitive with that of more advantaged students. Half of all public schools in the United States now receive Title I funding.

Title II of the ESEA supported school libraries and the acquisition of textbooks and instructional materials. It also funded preschool programs. States and school districts use Title II funds to recruit, prepare, and develop teachers and school administrators. As such, the purpose of Title II is to increase the number, quality, and effectiveness of teachers, principals, and other school leaders to improve student academic achievement, especially for low-income and minority students. Title III initially provided matching grants for supplementary education centers and, more generally, was the innovation component of the ESEA. It was later expanded into the Adult Education Act of 1966. This title offered additional services to bolster school attendance; it also mandated educational programming and special education services to be provided even in rural and remote areas. Two amendments to Title III in 1968, the Bilingual Education Act and the Education of the Handicapped Act, altered it so that federal funds supplement state funds for language instruction educational programs (which support students for whom English is not their first language or home language). These new developments help students learning English to achieve academic goals like other students. English language learners require specialized or modified instruction to suit their backgrounds in both English classes and their other academic courses, which are generally taught in English.

Title IV provided $100 million for educational research and training. This funding has continued across all of the subsequent iterations and has been modified along the way to provide additional funds. Title V supplemented grants to state departments of education, under the original purpose of reforming interactions between local and state educational systems. Under the title, local reforms were to parallel reforms at the state level. It also instituted support programs for libraries, scientific research, and improved teacher performance. Gifted programs, foreign language study, physical education, the arts, and the overall mental health care of students all also received money from the federal government. Title VI provided definitions and limitations related to the law for the purposes of later interpretation and implementation.

Title VII of the ESEA was added during the first reauthorization; in 1968, this title became the Bilingual Education Act. The original act left districts much room for interpretation, so not all school districts actually provided the services it outlined. The targeted schools were to provide English instruction in unison with students' native language. Some lawmakers later wanted to amend the law to view bilingualism as an asset instead of a deficit. However, many states struggled with the act and pushed for an English-only movement, with their schools taking an English immersion approach. One of the more notable examples is California's Proposition 227 in 1998, which replaced the state's bilingual education programs with 1-year English immersion programs. However, extensive research revealed no clear evidence to support superiority of this English learners instructional approach over others (American Institutes for Research and WestEd 2006). The Obama administration, as a result, pushed states to evaluate closely the academic progress of English learners. Since then, states have been held accountable for students' achievement and progress, employing bilingual programs where appropriate.

The initial years of the ESEA brought about many issues and debates related to federal funding and federal-state-local relations. The political climate of the country around and beyond the issue of education was tumultuous, and even though Title I proved valuable, people remained unhappy with inequities in how students from low-income families were receiving education.

The Times They've Been A-Changin': U.S. Education Policy Since 1965

It should be apparent that the ESEA of 1965 began a behemoth shift in education policy and funding. Some of the twists and turns during its reauthorizations over the decades are worth pointing out. For example, Congress enacted the Education Amendments of 1972, altering the ESEA. The new legislation, commonly known as Title IX, is a comprehensive federal law that protects students from sex-based discrimination in schools and other federally funded programs.

More than a decade later, the spotlight on education shifted its focus toward language learning in the classroom. In 1984, the ESEA was again amended under the Reagan administration, emphasizing bilingual education programming in Title II of the amendment. Title IV incorporated the Women's Educational Equity Amendments of 1984 as a successor of sorts to what Title IX had begun. Title V focused on the Indian Education Amendments of 1984, which expanded educational services for Native Americans. The Emergency Immigrant Education Act of 1984, affixed to Title VI, promoted English language instruction and other bilingual services.

The NCLB Act of 2001, as mentioned in the section "Elementary and Secondary Education Act of 1965," was an alteration of the ESEA under the administration of President George W. Bush. It favored school choice; individual liberties; and equal, universal compliance. It also sought to improve educational outcomes for some students with disabilities. Additionally, military recruiters were also now allowed to meet with eleventh and twelfth graders on school grounds. However, despite some positive outcomes, the act allowed states to lower their educational standards, leading them to focus on punishing failure over rewarding successes and on test scores rather than personal growth. The act encouraged schools to provide general interventions rather than individualized ones, and its mandate of compliance was ambitious and difficult to meet. The resulting punitive measures detracted from, rather than advanced, the act's own goals of equity.

President Obama reauthorized the ESEA in December of 2015 as the Every Student Succeeds Act. States now had flexibility when instituting some of the more unwieldy provisions of the law, leading to a wide range of implementations, with varying degrees of success. Each state must now show that it has adopted some particular standards and assessments, supported those schools most in need with the largest achievement gaps, and, on the district level, supported teachers' and principals' evaluations. In general terms, the Every Student Succeeds Act restored state and local control of education.

Changes again were made during President Donald J. Trump's administration. The Tax Cuts and Jobs Act expanded school choice. This allowed parents to use up to $10,000 from a 529 education savings account (designed to save for college tax free) to cover K–12 tuition costs at the public, private, or religious school of their choice. Some of his administration's policies took action to promote technical education as well. President Trump signed into law the Strengthening Career and Technical Education for the 21st Century Act, which provides more than 13 million students with high-quality vocational education and extends more than $1.3 billion each year to states for critical workforce development programs. Federal education policy will undoubtedly continue to evolve.

How the ESEA Influenced Mental Health

Both Esther Brown and Oliver Brown improved the mental health of Americans, and they did so by engaging the political process with determination and perseverance as everyday Americans with a passion for the pursuit of educational equality. Although it might not have been portrayed or even recognized as a mental health law, the ESEA strove to improve educational quality and educational equality which would improve mental health. The environments in which people learn, at all ages, directly and indirectly affect their health and well-being. This includes their mental health. In adulthood, those with less education are at greater risk for poor health in general (Johnson-Lawrence et al. 2017; Zajacova and Lawrence 2018), in part because they hold less secure jobs with less optimal pay. The higher one's education is, the lower one's rate of chronic diseases is. Moreover, effective education requires not only the attainment of academic skills but also important life skills such as healthy relationships, social support, and coping mechanisms, as well as understanding the meaning of work, self-regulation and control, and frustration tolerance. If we do not learn these important psychological and social skills at an early age, we are more prone to depression, anxiety, hostility, and feelings of hopelessness. In turn, these negative and harmful emotions affect our ability to cope with stress and can contribute to preventable mental and physical illnesses.

Most children in the United States receive their education in public primary and secondary schools. It is our duty to ensure that these environments are safe and health promoting, along with being fair and equitable as students learn. Through these steps, students will attain a higher quality of life in adulthood. Better education results in greater earnings, more opportunity to live in a safe environment, improved interpersonal relationships, greater preparation for parenting, richer social networks, and improved overall quality of life. In turn, these enhanced opportunities all lead to better physical and mental health. Low education is therefore one of the many and major social determinants of mental health (Powers 2015).

Poor education has been shown to affect mental health in many direct and indirect ways. For example, less schooling is directly related to health risk conditions such as smoking (Cao et al. 2018) and being overweight (Cohen et al. 2013). Higher educational level, above and beyond personal income, may also protect against becoming overweight or obese. Therefore, to prevent these significant health outcomes, we must focus on enhancing education. Furthermore, part of education's mission should be to support preventive efforts for all students in the school system. Consistent with the earlier link between area-level poverty and poor education, schools within low-socioeconomic-status communities often have a higher student-to-teacher ratio, a poorer quality of instruction, and a lack of adequate academic resources. All of these influence cognitive, social, and language development.

The social and mental health impacts of enhancing education extend back to the preschool years. Returning back to early childhood, the Head Start program continues to be the federally funded, locally implemented program to provide low-income preschoolers with education and health services. Since 1965, more than 30 million children and their low-income parents have received educational, social, health, and nutritional services through Head Start. In 1994, Head Start was expanded to create Early Head Start to include even younger children from birth to age 3. The Head Start budget remains too small to serve all in need, despite many studies showing improvements in domains such as higher test scores, higher high school graduation rates, fewer arrests, and higher lifetime earnings (Whitmore Schanzenbach and Bauer 2016).

Status of the War on Poverty

This story of education policy in the 1960s obviously coincided with the larger War on Poverty that was being waged. Scholars and historians still debate the actual effects of the War on Poverty (Sheffield and Rector 2014). Did it actually decrease poverty? Federal programs under this overarching policy initiative did help the poor overall, and the poverty rate actually decreased from 26% in 1967 to about 11% in 2020 (Statista 2021). The "war" began in 1964, and data collection began in 1967, leaving a gap of knowledge about its early effects. Most people believe poverty would have increased if the government programs described here had not been implemented. Food stamps (later renamed SNAP) alone kept 4 million people out of poverty. Social Security is a bigger program still. A few decades later, the Earned Income Tax Credit and other refundable credits assisted even more families. Not only did Medicare and Medicaid increase access to health care; they helped to lower poverty by reducing out-of-pocket medical costs. The Job Corps programs not only helped to ameliorate poverty but also reduced rates of incarceration, arrests, and conviction and increased rates of employment, earnings, and time spent employed (Schochet et al. 2008). However, many critics of the War on Poverty have charged that the most efficient ways to get people out of poverty are not to establish welfare programs but to create economic growth and reduce government dependency. Yet others say these varied programs for housing, education and job training, and family counseling should be better coordinated with each other to work best. The debate will go on.

Future of Improved and Equal Access to Education

It is difficult to identify ways in which expanded educational programs for everyone could ever be harmful. Along with a domestic agenda to reduce poverty and expand educational opportunities for all, increased financial aid to schools and training for those without adequate skills or education could advance the work force. There are a number of ongoing debates, which will undoubtedly inform further policy change.

Some believe a *track* system (e.g., a science track, an English/history track, an arts track, a vocational track), which some other countries have, could be feasible in the United States and would build on students' strengths and interests. This array of options might offer more possibilities for students with certain disabilities or with specific skill sets. Under this system, all students would take basic core classes and would then be able to take more advanced classes within the specific tracks. Not every student benefits from several years of foreign language classes or advanced math, for example, but others desire them and excel in such classes.

Socioemotional learning is also discussed as being as critical as academic pursuits. Along with specialized knowledge and skills that tracks might provide, students must learn key life skills: how to balance a bank account, do basic tax work, apply for a loan, build credit, interview and get a job, and so on. More self-care classes are also necessary. Because self-control and emotional health are key for success, we must teach students how to handle stress, depression, anxiety, and bullies, as well as about relationship building. Suicide prevention within schools is also critical. Suicide is the third leading cause of death in young people between ages 10 and 24 years. The suicide rate in children has increased dramatically since 2007 (Curtin and Heron 2019); some people feel that the rise may be partly related to the use of smartphones and other electronic devices.

The most important question in school should not be "Is this going to be on the test?" Building self-confidence, critical thinking abilities, and effective communication skills, rather than just good grades and test results, should be primary goals. Too often, students cram to memorize for tests rather than steadily moving toward understanding concepts and solving problems. The word *education* comes from a Latin word meaning *to train*, itself derived from the homonym *educo*, which means *to draw forth* or *bring out*. Schools should encourage students to draw forth and develop their natural abilities and strengths and to not be afraid to do so. Each student's passion should be brought out and nurtured. In school, too often, things are "put in" instead.

Many poor or otherwise disadvantaged young adults cannot attend college right out of high school; as such, they go directly to work and figure
out their interests much later, if ever. It would behoove the United States
to provide higher education opportunities for these individuals at a later
stage. Title I funds, from the original ESEA and the newest iterations,
could be used toward higher education well into college. An expansion of
community college opportunities would likely help millions. Universal free
community college has recently been deliberated and proposed (Saul and
Goldstein 2021).

Policies related to school choice continue to be deliberated. In May 2017
President Donald J. Trump's administration restored the D.C. Opportunity
Scholarship Program, the only federally funded school choice program in
the nation, which allows disadvantaged students from low-income families
in Washington, D.C., to attend schools of their choice. K–12 students can
choose the right education fit for each of them to better meet their learning
needs and improve their chance for future success. Scholarships go to students in families with an average annual income less than $27,000, with
more than 90% self-identifying as Black or Hispanic/Latino. Although just
a demonstration in one city, the scholarship has allowed more than 1,500
students in the D.C. area to attend private schools of their choice. For those
supporting school choice, the idea is that competition will improve overall
school performance in a community where school choice is given. Issues
around school choice and access to and funding for charter schools remain
hot topics in education policy, with some people concerned that these programs strip resources from public school systems, making underresourced
systems even worse.

There continues to be room for substantial policy improvement in the
arena of education. For example, despite the promise of the ESEA of 1965,
racial/ethnic school segregation has gotten worse since the 1970s (García
2020). The implications of this are concerning and suggest structural unintended consequences that undoubtedly interfere with the original promise of
the ESEA, and these consequences must be understood and addressed.

There are also reasons for hope about the future of education in the
United States. Today, high school graduations and college attendance are
both at an all-time high. Dropout rates are at an all-time low. However, the
U.S. public education system still has a long way to go. The original ESEA
was a great beginning toward helping the United States achieve improved
and equal education for all. As such, because educational quality, educational equality, and education attainment are powerful determinants of
physical health and mental health (Powers 2015), the nation's health has
been improved by it. Even though it has changed dramatically throughout

the years, its provisions still offer a powerful means through which students can attain better education and thus ultimately better mental health.

The times really did change during the 1960s. Many of the decade's events have dramatically influenced what is happening in the United States today, and the American educational system is different for it. As the times keep a-changin', we must continue to search for better ways to serve the mental health of the nation, and that must start in the incubator of its future, the school.

References

American Institutes for Research; WestEd: Effects of the Implementation of Proposition 227 on the Education of English Learners, K–12: Findings From a Five-Year Evaluation. San Francisco, CA, WestEd, January 24, 2006. Available at: www2.wested.org/www-static/online_pubs/227Reportb.pdf. Accessed June 21, 2022.

Cao P, Jeon J, Tam J, et al: Smoking disparities by level of educational attainment in the United States, 1966 to 2015. Tobacco Induced Diseases 16(suppl 1):A899, 2018

Cohen AK, Rai M, Abrams B: Educational attainment and obesity: a systematic review. Obes Rev14(12):989–1005, 2013 23889851

Curtin SC, Heron M: Death rates due to suicide and homicide among persons aged 10–24: United States, 2000–2017. NCHS Data Brief 352:1–8, 2019 31751202

Ganzel B: Farming in the 1950s and 60s: education in rural America. York, NE, Wessels Living History Farm, 2007. Available at: https://livinghistoryfarm.org/farminginthe50s/life_12.html. Accessed November 18, 2021.

García E: Schools are still segregated, and Black children are paying a price. Washington, DC, Economic Policy Institute, February 12, 2020. Available at: www.epi.org/publication/schools-are-still-segregated-and-black-children-are-paying-a-price. Accessed November 19, 2021.

Holland A, Andre T: Participation in extracurricular activities in secondary school: what is known, what needs to be known? Rev Educ Res 57(4):437–466, 1987

Jayne GD: Little Rock Nine. Encyclopedia Britannica, March 11, 2020. Available at: www.britannica.com/topic/Little-Rock-Nine. Accessed September 3, 2021.

Johnson-Lawrence V, Zajacova A, Sneed R: Education, race/ethnicity, and multimorbidity among adults aged 30–64 in the National Health Interview Survey. SSM Popul Health 3:366–372, 2017 29349230

Katz MS, Tucker SB: A pioneer in civil rights: Esther Brown and the South Park desegregation case of 1948. Kans Hist 18(4):234–247, 1995

Klein A: No Child Left Behind: an overview. Education Week, 2015. Available at: www.edweek.org/policy-politics/no-child-left-behind-an-overview/2015/04. Accessed November 19, 2021.

Linder DO: Meet the Browns: Esther Brown and the Oliver Brown family. Kansas City, University of Missouri–Kansas City School of Law, 2011. Available at: http://law2.umkc.edu/faculty/projects/ftrials/brownvboard/meetthebrowns.html. Accessed November 18, 2021.

National Park Services: Rev. Oliver L. Brown: Brown v. Board of Education National Historic Site. National Park Service, 2021. Available at: www.nps.gov/people/oliver-brown.htm. Accessed November 18, 2021.

Powers R: Poor education, in The Social Determinants of Mental Health. Edited by Compton MT, Shim RS. Washington, DC, American Psychiatric Association Publishing, 2015, pp 77–98

Saul S, Goldstein D: Biden directs education funding to community colleges, a key lifeline. The New York Times, May 2, 2021. Available at: www.nytimes.com/2021/04/28/us/politics/biden-education-community-college.html. Accessed February 16, 2022.

Schochet PZ, Burghardt J, McConnell S: Does Jobs Corps work? Impact findings from the National Job Corps Study. American Economic Review 98(5):1864–1886, 2008

Sheffield R, Rector R: The War on Poverty after 50 years. Washington, DC, The Heritage Foundation, September 15, 2014. Available at: www.heritage.org/poverty-and-inequality/report/the-war-poverty-after-50-years. Accessed September 3, 2021.

Statista: Poverty rate in the United States from 1990 to 2020. New York, Statista, 2021. Available at: www.statista.com/statistics/200463/us-poverty-rate-since-1990. Accessed November 19, 2021.

U.S. Department of Agriculture: Education. Washington, DC, Economic Research Service, 2021. Available at: https://data.ers.usda.gov/reports.aspx?ID=17829. Accessed November 18, 2021.

U.S. Department of Education: Supporting school reform by leveraging federal funds in a schoolwide program: non-regulatory guidance. Washington, DC, U.S. Department of Agriculture, September 2016. Available at: https://www2.ed.gov/policy/elsec/leg/essa/essaswpguidance9192016.pdf. Accessed November 19, 2021.

U.S. Department of Education: Every Student Succeeds Act (ESSA). Washington, DC, U.S. Department of Education, 2022. Available at: www.ed.gov/essa?src=rn. Accessed February 15, 2022.

Virginia Museum of History and Culture: Massive Resistance. Richmond, Virginia Museum of History and Culture, 2021. Available at: https://virginiahistory.org/learn/historical-book/chapter/massive-resistance. Accessed November 18, 2021.

Whitmore Schanzenbach D, Bauer L: The long-term impact of the Head Start program. Washington, DC, Brookings Institution, August 19, 2016. Available at: www.brookings.edu/research/the-long-term-impact-of-the-head-start-program. Accessed November 19, 2021.

Zajacova A, Lawrence EM: The relationship between education and health: reducing disparities through a contextual approach. Annu Rev Public Health 39(1):273–289, 2018 29328865

8 | Remodeling and Breaking New Ground

The Housing and Urban Development Act of 1965

Jacob M. Izenberg, M.D.
Brie A. Garner, M.P.H.
Andrew T. Turk, M.D., A.M.

A Day in Watts

Until he was pulled over by police that evening, Marquette Frye must have assumed August 11, 1965, would be a day like any other in the Watts neighborhood of Los Angeles, California. As officers prepared to arrest Mr. Frye on suspicion of drunk driving, his mother, Rena Price, was drawn out of her nearby home and tried to intervene. Precisely what happened in the next few moments is unclear, but the situation became heated. Ms. Price and Mr. Frye were both assaulted, and outrage over police brutality quickly spread. Soon, a pent-up store of collective anger erupted into the Watts Rebellion (Folkart 1986). In the end, 34 people were dead (Gershon 2016). A week after the protests, Martin Luther King Jr. flew to Los Angeles. Speaking about the riots, he pleaded for nonviolent political action. However, observing the conditions that had led to so much frustration and anger, he acknowledged, "The economic deprivation, social isolation, inadequate housing, and general despair of thousands of Negroes teeming in Northern and Western ghettos are the ready seeds which give birth to tragic expressions of violence" (Martin Luther King, Jr., Research and Education Institute 2018). Watts was one such "Western ghetto," located in the heart of a mid-twentieth-century Los Angeles that although relatively young as a metropolis, was rather typical in at least one way: it was deeply segregated by race. Black families were excluded from white neighborhoods by force of law and vigilantism alike. The neighborhoods into which they were able to move were cut off from financing and investment, politically marginalized, isolated from other parts of the city, fractured, and underserviced. Dr. King saw and spoke to the injustice of these conditions.

In 1968, the so-called Kerner Commission was tasked with taking stock of the late 1960s civil unrest that scarred numerous American cities, including Los Angeles. The commission recognized the importance of racial injustice across a range of policy domains, with housing prominent among them, and in their report (Kerner Commission 1968), the members laid out some key facts about housing in America just before the Watts Rebellion. In the decades leading up to 1965, Black Americans were excluded from white neighborhoods through discrimination in virtually every aspect of the housing market, limiting their options to relatively few areas. Excluded from most neighborhoods and from the generous programs making home ownership affordable to working-class white families, Black families were vulnerable to exploitation by landlords who often subdivided units while nevertheless charging exorbitant rents. As a result, Black renters, already facing economic exclusion and labor market discrimination, were nevertheless more likely to be paying *higher* prices for housing than white renters; this was for dwellings that were disproportionately undermaintained, lacking in essentials such as plumbing and heating, and overcrowded. Local governments, which were less likely to enforce housing codes in minority neighborhoods, effectively looked the other way (Kerner Commission 1968).

What was the federal government doing to ameliorate this situation? The commission members criticized the woefully inadequate housing programs for low-income Americans, particularly when compared with the dynamo of suburban middle-class housing construction:

> Federal programs have been able to do comparatively little to provide housing for the disadvantaged. In the 31-year history of subsidized federal housing, only about 800,000 units have been constructed, with recent production averaging about 50,000 units a year. By comparison, over a pe-

riod of only 3 years longer, FHA insurance guarantees have made possible the construction of over 10 million middle- and upper-income units. (Kerner Commission 1968, pp. 259–260)

Indeed, for decades after the inception of the Federal Housing Administration (FHA), it frequently mandated the exclusion of Black residents from the neighborhoods and developments in which it was offering the sort of insurance guarantees described in the above passage (Figure 8–1) (Rothstein 2017).

Coincidentally, the day before Marquette Frye's arrest precipitated the Watts Rebellion, President Lyndon B. Johnson signed into law one of the most expansive federal housing bills to date: the Housing and Urban Development Act of 1965. Like all federal housing policy, the law's legacy is complex. At its core, however, it was seeking to address one of the very issues the Kerner Commission report would later emphasize: a lack of affordable housing for low-income Americans.

The Great Society and the Urban Crisis

Johnson assumed the office of the presidency on November 27, 1963. The Watts Rebellion was nearly 2 years in the future, but the shocking assassination of John F. Kennedy 5 days earlier presaged the turbulent period ahead. The serious problems facing American cities were already apparent. Well underway was the explosive suburban growth that excluded Black people and encouraged *white flight* from urban areas. Meanwhile, government programs ostensibly designed to remake cities in a modern, automobile-centric twentieth century vision were, in fact, obliterating otherwise vibrant communities of color, replacing them with expanses of concrete, civic areas, barren office plazas, and freeways. As the Kerner Commission (1968) noted, the construction of federally subsidized housing had been anemic, and some of the flagship projects of the 1950s were already falling into disrepair. Although the Watts Rebellion and the episodes of social unrest that followed are often viewed collectively as a watershed moment for the urban crisis in America, in reality, it was a crisis decades in the making.

When Johnson began his first and only full term in office in January 1965, he brought with him an overwhelmingly Democratic Congress and a mandate to press ahead with Kennedy's progressive agenda, a major focus of which was poverty. The problem of poverty in American society was not new, but after nearly a decade of relative neglect under Eisenhower, the issue was getting attention again. Indeed, in service of this cause, Johnson declared a War on Poverty at the start of his administration (Brauer 1982) and embarked on a program that ultimately took the form of the Great Society,

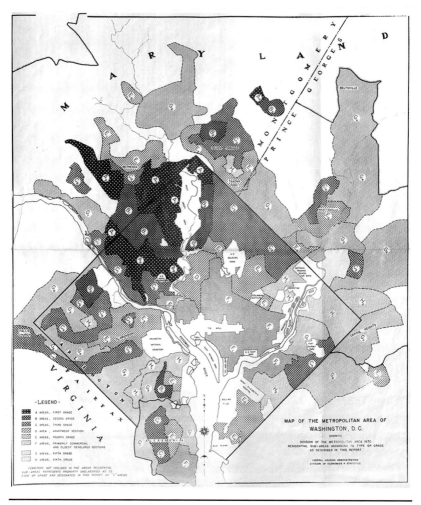

FIGURE 8–1.   Residential subareas, Federal Housing Administration (FHA), 1937.

This map produced by the FHA was used for housing mortgage lending and investment. It assigns letter grades to every block in Washington, D.C., to define the value of each residential area for housing investment. The code for this map explicitly uses race as a criterion and assigns lower grades for residential subareas for Black communities. Similar to the redlining maps of the 1930s, the FHA maps are just one example of the many forms of housing discrimination.

Source.   Housing Market Analysis, Washington, D.C., July 1937. Federal Housing Administration Statistics, August 5, 1937. Research and Statistics Division, Records Relating to Housing Market Analyses 1935–1942, Box 17, RG 31, National Archives. D.C. Policy Center: "Mapping Segregation in D.C. 2019." Available at: www.dcpolicycenter.org/publications/mapping-segregation-fha. Accessed June 7, 2022.

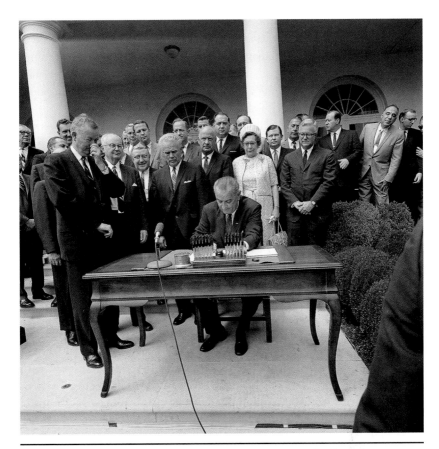

FIGURE 8-2.   **President Lyndon B. Johnson signing the Housing and Urban Development Act in the White House Rose Garden on August 10, 1965.**
Source.   LBJ Presidential Library, Austin, TX. Available at: www.lbjlibrary.org/object/photo/signing-housing-and-urban-development-act-0. Accessed February 16, 2022. Public domain.

the largest raft of federal domestic policy since the New Deal. A cornerstone of this effort was addressing housing insecurity and the plight of disinvested urban neighborhoods (Figure 8–2) (von Hoffman 2009).

Robert Weaver and the Tensions in American Policy

Robert Weaver (Figure 8–3) was born into a middle-class Washington, D.C., family, one whose story was arguably not typical for Black Americans of the era but placed it among the "small but vibrant black elite in Washington" (Pritchett 2008). Weaver's great-grandfather was a former slave in North Carolina who had managed to purchase his freedom with earnings from carpentry work. His grandfather was the first Black graduate of Harvard's dentistry program, and by the mid-1930s, Robert Weaver held a doctorate in economics from Harvard (Pritchett 2008).

At the time Weaver earned his degree, President Franklin D. Roosevelt was in the midst of remaking the American economic system through the New Deal. Although most New Deal policies allowed or even encouraged segregation, Roosevelt did convene a so-called Black Cabinet, a group of Black advisers on New Deal economic and policy issues relating to Black Americans, and Weaver started his career as a member of that group (Pritchett 2008). After continuing in government and foundation work related to housing, including, eventually, as the New York State rent commissioner, Weaver returned to the federal government and joined the Kennedy administration as the administrator of the House and Home Financing Agency, a precursor to the Department of Housing and Urban Development (HUD).

When HUD was established in 1965, Weaver became its first secretary and earned the distinction of being the first Black American to lead a cabinet-level department. He had earned the role by being at the forefront of the Johnson administration's efforts on housing, often working closely with liberal housing advocates on the details of legislation, advocating for progressive reforms, and testifying in Congress to help advance the Kennedy and Johnson administrations' agendas (von Hoffman 2009). His contributions to the development of Great Society housing and urban policy were enormous. Weaver was an advocate for civil rights, including fair housing, who collaborated closely with and contributed to organizations such as the National Association for the Advancement of Colored People (NAACP) (Pritchett 2008).

Despite his advocacy, Weaver's legacy is not without complication. In a 1960 paper, he wrote,

> Revitalizing cities is more than a real estate operation. It involves reaching and assisting the residents of slums and blighted areas, learning more about them and society's attitudes toward them in the process. In doing so, we will doubtless come to appreciate that some of their values—although strikingly different from those of the dominant groups in our society—are not only utilitarian but worthy of emulation. Many of their patterns of behavior, while unacceptable to the majority, may well be compatible with successful urban living; others will require mediation. (Weaver 1960, p. 39).

In this passage, Weaver revealed a fundamental problem with liberal urban policy in the mid-twentieth century. Although not explicitly stated by

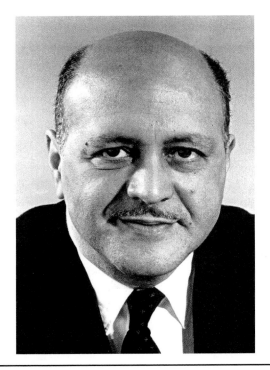

FIGURE 8–3. Official portrait of Robert Weaver, Secretary of the Department of Housing and Urban Development.
Source. Department of Housing and Urban Development, Washington, D.C. Public domain. Available at: https://catalog.archives.gov/id/24070810. Accessed May 15, 2022.

Weaver, the "residents of slums and blighted areas" were predominately Black and had limited alternative options thanks to exclusion from white neighborhoods (Rothstein 2017). The "slums" and "blight" in which they lived were the product of redlining (the practice of restricting financing and investment in neighborhoods of color) and other forms of racialized disinvestment (Fullilove 2005). Weaver's writing, at least in the passage above, positions these urban dwellers in *juxtaposition* to society, rather than as part of it. Viewing Black city dwellers as part of a problem that "society" needed to fix was part of the intellectual foundation of urban renewal, the federal policy that funded the demolition of disinvested urban neighborhoods with the effect of obliterating and displacing hundreds of thriving communities (Fullilove 2005). Weaver understood this legacy, yet as House and Home Financing Agency administrator and then HUD secretary, he oversaw the program and frequently found himself defending it (Pritchett 2008). On the other hand, Weaver's words also acknowledge the ingenuity, adaptation, and creativity of urban life at a time when many policy makers and urban leaders viewed marginalized urban neighborhoods as landscapes of invariable degeneracy. Weaver's efforts to temper some of the worst excesses of urban renewal presumably reflected this sort of thinking. Some of these efforts would bear fruit when, in 1965, Johnson tasked Weaver with engineering the flagship housing legislation of the Great Society.

Politics of Rent Subsidies

After Congress passed the Housing and Urban Development Act of 1965, Johnson held a press conference. He could have talked about any number of things; after all, his administration had just advanced a massive piece of legislation with a broad array of provisions—in effect the largest federal housing bill to date. But Johnson emphasized just a couple of highlights, including a program of rent subsidies and a grant program for low-income families to rehabilitate their housing (Semple 1965). It is not surprising that Johnson would have wanted to address these hard-won provisions in particular. Indeed, the rent subsidy program produced enough resistance to nearly sink the bill in a Congress generally friendly to the Johnson agenda. Although the subsidy programs were ultimately somewhat narrow and short-lived, they would set the tone for American low-income housing policy to a degree that could not have been fully understood at the time.

In effect, the program worked like this: First, the FHA insured mortgages for new low-income housing projects built or owned by private, nonprofit entities such as limited-dividend corporations, building cooperatives, churches, and labor unions. Second, for families accepted as tenants by these groups, the law empowered HUD to provide subsidies to cover the difference between an affordable cost to the family and a fair market rent for the unit, such that the family would pay one-fourth of its income, and HUD would pay the difference to the owner (Biles 2000). This endeavor aligned with traditional approaches to low-income housing assistance programs, which had generally been designed and implemented in order to promote new construction. The subsidy provision authorized $150 million in contracts over a 4-year period, which advocates estimated would facilitate construction of 375,000 new homes, predominantly in the form of apartments (Semple 1965). Another section of the bill, the so-called Section 23 Leased Housing Program, authorized local public housing authorities (PHAs) to identify suitable units on the private market that could serve as low-income housing, lease those apartments, and then sublease them to eligible tenants at a rent comparable to traditional (i.e., government built and operated) public housing.

As with much of housing policy, the design, scope, and, in many ways, limitations of the rent supplementation program were the product of compromise around, for example, the income range for eligibility and the extent of local control (Schwartz 2014). This compromise in part came from the fierce political battle over the program. Weaver himself did not originally support rent subsidies, tending to favor traditional public housing instead (Pritchett 2008). In fact, these supplements had something of a conservative origin. Going back to the 1930s, the U.S. Chamber of Commerce and housing industry leaders had pitched rent supplementation as an alternative to public housing (von Hoffman 2009). This pedigree concerned some liberals, but by the 1960s, the idea of rent supplements had gained traction among many people on the left. Weaver himself had become an advocate, recognizing that the political will to expand public housing construction had waned and coming to view rent subsidies as a way to expand the reach of housing support beyond the lowest-income families (von Hoffman 2009). The supplements also had the unspoken appeal of promising to reduce racial segregation by offering people of color more options in their housing choices (Pritchett 2008); although not widely discussed at the time, this would later come to be viewed as one of the more appealing aspects of this approach to housing (Schwartz 2014).

Johnson also underscored a generous provision in the bill providing grants of up to $1,500 (roughly $12,000 in 2020 dollars) intended for rehabilitation of properties inhabited by low-income residents. The subsidy and grant plans thus complemented one another, according to Johnson, enabling "the construction and rehabilitation of housing for older adults and for families of low income—the people who live in the most wretched conditions" (Semple 1965).

Emboldened by divisions among various lobbying groups and marshaling Cold War anxieties, the bill's congressional opponents laid into the rent subsidy program, arguing that it "smacked of socialism" (Semple 1965). Deploying a common line of conservative reasoning, political opponents worried that the bill would undermine Americans' incentives to improve their housing conditions through hard work or to strive toward home ownership (Krock 1965). They also used thinly veiled language such as *socioeconomic integration* to attack the subsidy program's potential to offer Black families a chance to afford living in wealthier, predominately white areas (von Hoffman 2009). These debates overshadowed much of the rest of the extensive bill and, as noted, nearly derailed it. Ultimately, however, proponents were able to muscle the bill through Congress, partly by compromising on issues such as the income threshold for rent subsidy eligibility (von Hoffman 2009). After the bill's passage, Johnson foreshadowed what would come to be a major role for the private sector and touted incentives and opportunities for industry, arguing that "private builders will be able to move into the low-income housing field which they have not been able to penetrate or to serve effectively in the past" (Semple 1965).

Some aspects of the final law were championed by Republicans, includ-ing features that supported business owners and military service members (Semple 1965). One such measure increased availability of federal housing benefits to members of the military and those affected by military facility closures. In the Senate, Republican Leverett Saltonstall of Massachusetts introduced an amendment that assured timely public hearings to commu-nities affected by HUD programs, added on behalf of businesses potentially displaced or otherwise affected by urban renewal initiatives.

Housing and Urban Development Act of 1965

The Housing and Urban Development Act of 1965 (hereafter referred to as the Housing Act) was a massive law. An omnibus bill, the law's 11 titles contained a range of housing- and urban-development-related provisions; only a selection of key provisions is given here (Table 8–1). Title I of the Housing Act is of particular interest because it focused on financial assis-tance to vulnerable families, including low-income groups, older adults, those with disabilities, victims of natural disasters, those displaced by other means, and those living in "substandard housing" (Housing and Urban De-velopment Act 1965). Some of Title I's most noteworthy provisions include the rent subsidy provisions detailed in the section "Politics of Rent Subsi-dies": Section 101, the rent supplement plan, and Section 103, often re-ferred to as the Section 23 Leased Housing Program in reference to the sections amended in the original 1937 Housing Act. These plans provided the first significant federal effort to leverage the private market for public housing by either contracting with nonprofit organizations willing to build housing or offering funds to help local PHAs broker and subsidize rental arrangements on the private market. Several other sections of Title I of-fered important supports to vulnerable populations at risk of housing insta-bility or displacement. Section 104 was another significant development in housing policy whereby the definition of an eligible "family" was modified to include older adults and disabled individuals, even if they lived alone. An-other key part of Title I, Section 106, authorized local agencies to issue grants of up to $1,500 to families in designated urban renewal areas making $3,000 or less annually (just over $12,000 and $24,000 in 2020 dollars, re-spectively; for consistency, all contemporary figures will be given in 2020 amounts) with the goal of making those homes meet the standards neces-sary to avoid their destruction. This provision was, at least in theory, one of the first federally sponsored efforts to empower residents of urban re-newal areas to escape from wholesale neighborhood demolition.

TABLE 8–1. Summary of selected key provisions of the Housing and Urban Development Act of 1965

	Title name	Description	Key provisions	Significance
Title I	Special Provisions for Disadvantaged Persons	Financial assistance to vulnerable families (e.g., low-income households, older adults, those with disabilities, victims of natural disasters or displaced individuals, and those living in "substandard housing")	1. Section 101: rent supplement plan 2. Section 103: leased housing program 3. Section 104: changed definition of eligible "family" to include single older adults and disabled individuals 4. Section 106: grants for families in urban renewal areas for home renovations in an effort to avoid neighborhood demolition	Provided the first significant federal effort to leverage the private market for public housing through the following: 1. Contracting with nonprofit organizations to build housing 2. Providing funds to local public housing authorities to broker and subsidize rents in the private market
Title II	FHA Insurance Operations	Updated federal mortgage insurance program	Section 201	Established federal mortgage insurance program for land development
Title III	Urban Renewal	Revised urban renewal program: 1. Maintained authorization for "slum clearance" 2. Code enforcement and rehabilitation loans for the repair of and investment in deteriorating neighborhoods	Section 305: relocation of individuals displaced from urban renewal areas	Maintained slum clearance but offered some additional funding to avoid demolition and relocate displaced families

TABLE 8–1. Summary of selected key provisions of the Housing and Urban Development Act of 1965 *(continued)*

	Title name	Description	Key provisions	Significance
Title IV	Compensation of Condemnees	Established provisions to compensate households displaced under eminent domain	Sections 401–404	Provided some additional mitigation of harms from urban renewal
Title V	Low-Rent Public Housing	Expanded public housing programs; authorized substantial additional funding for new public housing construction	Sections 501–507	Authorized significant new funds for public housing
Title VII	Community Facilities	Provided federal grants for public works	Section 703: grants for neighborhood facilities (e.g., recreation centers)	Created new funding for community investment
Title IX	Open-Space Land and Urban Beautification and Improvement	Provided federal grants for neighborhood beautification and improvement projects	Sections 901–908	Promoted investment in parks and conservation of urban green spaces and natural areas

Note. FHA=Federal Housing Administration.

Title II of the legislation primarily concerned updates of the federal mortgage insurance program. Title III of the law made several revisions to urban renewal, largely keeping in place authorization for the federal policy of neighborhood demolition and displacement in the name of "slum clearance." However, along with the Title I rehabilitation grants, some provisions of Title III offered a subtle nudge in a different direction—specifically, repair of and investment in deteriorating neighborhoods through code enforcement and rehabilitation loans. Other provisions included revisions to programs assisting in the relocation of families displaced by urban renewal and mandates that specific urban renewal projects be in accordance with local agencies' master plans. Title IV established provisions that sought to codify "fair" compensation for displacement under eminent domain (Housing and Urban Development Act 1965).

Title V of the Housing Act concerned the expansion of traditional public housing programs, including a sizable increase in the funding authorization for federally subsidized public housing and annual contributions to local PHAs, in effect authorizing roughly 240,000 new public housing units (von Hoffman 2009).

Several provisions of the law provided federal grants for the acquisition of land for sewer and water systems, as well as community facilities such as recreation centers. The law also provided increased funding for communities seeking to develop and maintain open spaces or engage in general beautification and other improvement projects. Finally, the Housing Act addressed a range of issues, including loans for rural housing, federal insurance programs, housing near military facilities, college housing construction loans, and grants for urban planning and research efforts. Many of these were revisions to earlier housing legislation that increased the dollar amounts available for various loan programs, insurance funds, grant-making authorities, and the like.

Placing the 1965 Housing Act Within the Lineage of Federal Housing Policy

Federal housing policy as we know it today grew out of the Great Depression housing crisis and the New Deal. Under President Franklin D. Roosevelt, the federal government created large housing agencies, got into the business of insuring and standardizing home mortgages, and, with the Housing Act of 1937, began a large-scale effort to build low-income public housing. The Housing Act of 1949 expanded these programs and launched the now infamous urban renewal program in earnest. The 1965 Housing Act, the focus of this chapter, was one of several laws to effectively expand on, revise, and add to this 1949 law. The 1968 Fair Housing Act (officially Title VIII of the Civil Rights Act of 1968) mandated nondiscrimination in housing. Building on programs pioneered in the 1965 Housing Act, the Housing and Community Development Act of 1974 created the rent subsidies programs for low-income families that are today popularly known as Section 8. In the 1990s, HOPE VI (an administrative initiative at HUD) sought to remake long-neglected federal housing projects in the image of mixed-income neighborhoods. Other developments in low-income housing policy came in the form of tax legislation, such as the development of the Low-Income Housing Tax Credit, a program to incentivize affordable housing construction through tax breaks, in the 1980s. An entire chapter could be written on the complex legacies of any one of these initiatives, and indeed, many have been the subjects of entire bodies of literature. Ultimately, none of them stand alone in the complex network of federal housing policy. That we focus on the 1965 Housing Act should not be taken to suggest it was the single most significant piece of legislation; its programs can be traced through generations of iterative policy making.

Over the past 80 years, virtually no part of federal housing law has escaped criticism, with good reason. For one thing, racism and segregation were baked into the major federal housing programs at their inception, leaving a legacy of residential discrimination, exclusion, and community displacement that persists to this day (Fullilove 2005; Rothstein 2017). The destructive force of urban renewal is also hard to overstate. This program—which was at the core of twentieth-century federal housing policy, including the 1965 Housing Act—tore through urban neighborhoods, particularly majority-Black areas, fracturing entire communities, reinforcing segregation, and ultimately hollowing out many once vibrant cities (Fullilove 2005). Later efforts were prone to perpetuate these wrongs, as demonstrated by the further displacement caused by many of the HOPE VI projects in the 1990s (Fullilove and Wallace 2011). Section 8, the heir to the rent supplement programs of the 1965 Housing Act, has itself had a mixed legacy, beset by excessive wait times and the vulnerability of voucher holders to discrimination and exclusion in the rental market (Mazzara 2017). These and other important critiques notwithstanding, the federal government has inarguably played a major role in providing housing to millions of the nation's most economically vulnerable. The 1965 Housing Act represented somewhat of a turning point in this direction in that it initiated federal rent subsidy policies, increased funding for traditional public housing, increased aid to vulnerable individuals, and pushed urban renewal more toward rehabilitation than simple wide-scale demolition of neighborhoods. Federal housing law must be considered in view of this massive, if deeply imperfect and frequently unjust, legacy. Indeed, many of the ideas for solving today's housing crisis have evolved, for better or for worse, from the policies of the twentieth century. Given the political realities of the U.S. system, it is likely that approaches to addressing the housing policy challenges of the next few decades will continue to build on these earlier efforts.

Impact of the Housing Act

Housing

In substantially increasing the authorized allocations to PHAs for the creation of low-income housing, the 1965 Housing Act marked a considerable federal recommitment to such efforts and created momentum for housing production that persisted through the end of the following decade. Despite a period of moratorium under the Nixon administration, the 1970s saw the largest growth in the stock of public housing of any decade before or since (Schwartz 2014). Public housing units of the sort described in this chapter were originally authorized by the 1937 Wagner-Steagall Act, but by the 1960s, many were viewed as failures. Public housing was, indeed, a deeply flawed program in many ways, subject to the racially discriminatory and exclusionary whims of local PHAs (Rothstein 2017). Projects were often cheaply built, and in part because of the fiscal approach to their upkeep—which relied primarily on rent—they were often poorly maintained (Schwartz 2014). They were frequently designed according to a modernist vision unconducive to community cohesion, safety, and well-being (Jacobs 1961). Such shortcomings were important and yielded the high-profile implosions (both figurative and literal) of several flagship projects, such as Pruitt-Igoe, a massive St. Louis complex so immediately beset by these problems that it was demolished only two decades after opening (von Hoffman 1996). Examples like these notwithstanding, it is also the case that much of the maligning of public housing is due to concerted political resistance on the part of actors ideologically and economically opposed to government-subsidized housing, resistance that often capitalized on high-profile failures or, in some cases, other political currents such as anti-communist sentiment (Parson 2016; von Hoffman 2010). The success of this agenda has established a popular narrative around the failure of public housing that contains some truth but is incomplete. Many public housing projects are scatter-site, low-rise developments that blend in with local neighborhoods and are managed by PHAs with 500 units or fewer (Schwartz 2014). Today, 1.8 million Americans have stable homes in public housing units (Center on Budget and Policy Priorities 2021). Furthermore, in part thanks to language in the 1965 Housing Act expanding protections for low-income older adults and disabled residents, members of these particularly vulnerable groups head more than half of the households in today's public housing today (Center on Budget and Policy Priorities 2021).

Although the 1965 Housing Act committed the government to significant new construction of federal housing, the act's once-controversial rent subsidy programs have, arguably, left an even more durable legacy, if a mixed one. The law allowed the federal government, for the first time, to subsidize—through several different mechanisms—the rental of private market housing for eligible families. It would ultimately be another decade before the advent of the so-called Section 8 programs that today make up the bulk of federal rental subsidies, but the 1965 provisions were the first of such efforts. With the decline in political support for large-scale public housing, these sorts of programs have grown in importance to the point where they have come to house considerably more Americans than does traditional public housing. Specifically, two large Section 8 programs subsidize the rents of recipients by making payments to landlords, ensuring that families pay no more than a set percentage of income in rent—the key distinction being whether the vouchers are portable (housing choice) or tied to a particular building (project based). Of the roughly 10 million individuals relying on some form of federal rental or housing assistance (including traditional public housing), roughly three-quarters are receiving Section 8 support: about 5 million people through the Housing Choice Voucher Program (Center on Budget and Policy Priorities 2017a) and about 2 million through Project-Based Rental Assistance (Center on Budget and Policy Priorities 2017b). The rent subsidy program that was passed under the 1965 Housing Act set the legal and policy precedent for these far larger programs, even though the subsidies in the 1965 law were ultimately small and never gained the funding or traction needed for widespread implementation.

If vouchers are a legacy of the 1965 Housing Act, that legacy is a complicated one. Although the programs are far larger than earlier subsidies, the success of today's voucher programs is still limited by underfunding and discrimination. Currently, because of chronic funding limitations and low supply, only one in four households eligible for housing choice vouchers receives them (Leopold et al. 2015; Scally et al. 2018). In many medium-to-large cities, individuals and families linger on voucher waitlists for periods measured in years or even decades (National Low Income Housing Coalition 2016). Worse, most eligible families are not even in the queue: currently, almost 3 million families are waiting to receive a voucher, but more than 9 million more are excluded because of waitlist caps and closures (Mazzara 2017). Even if a household manages to obtain a voucher, it has become increasingly difficult to find a landlord who will accept it (Bell et al. 2018). Although a growing number of states and municipalities have protections against discrimination based on source of income, federal law currently does not prohibit landlords from rejecting housing vouchers (Bell et al. 2018). It is also not uncommon to be denied housing assistance entirely because of a substance use disorder or a history of involvement in the criminal justice system (Curtis et al. 2013). Although rent subsidy programs have been instrumental in housing millions of Americans, these major problems underscore the fact that they have remained unable to even come close to meeting the need, at least thus far.

Urban Renewal

The 1965 Housing Act perpetuated the catastrophic federal program known as urban renewal, which originated with Title I of the Housing Act of 1949 and was sustained by the series of federal housing omnibus bills passed in subsequent decades. Urban renewal funded local efforts to seize, through eminent domain, swaths designated as "slums" or "blighted" areas, raze them, and redevelop the land for other uses. The program overwhelmingly targeted people of color, who comprised three-quarters of those displaced by the program's roughly 2,500 projects across nearly 1,000 American cities (Fullilove and Wallace 2011). The neighborhoods destroyed by urban renewal, typically in need of the very sort of investment denied them through decades of discriminatory policy, were, nevertheless, often vibrant and densely populated. In their place, cities erected countless faceless and uninhabitable infrastructure projects such as convention centers and malls and paved hundreds of miles of interstate highways. Much of this development was undertaken with little to no citywide planning to better meet the needs of inhabitants and in many cases left the weedy scars of incomplete efforts (Fullilove 2005; Jacobs 1961; Rothstein 2017). For those projects involving new housing, it was frequently not for former residents, who in many cases were instead relocated to the same massive public housing projects that would come to be seen as failures or to other parts of the city entirely, often creating new, worse slums. Urban renewal devastated inner-city communities of color, undermining community social cohesion and giving rise to a collective trauma that Dr. Mindy Fullilove has referred to as "root shock" (Fullilove 2005). The 1965 Housing Act did contain some incremental changes to urban renewal that appear to have been efforts to address a growing backlash against the program, such as the law's grants and loans for rehabilitation and its efforts to support code enforcement, which might, in theory, prevent neighborhoods from declining in the first place. However, the law generally left the practice intact and ignored the fact that urban renewal was a ready tool for municipal authorities eager to take land from communities of color and disperse residents (Fullilove 2005; Sugrue 1996).

Link Between Housing and Mental Health

There are many relationships between housing and mental health. Housing is, after all, the context in which so much of one's life occurs, and it is often the venue for what we consider essential—nourishment, safety, warmth and comfort, family ties and friendship, intimacy, education, and so much else. The home is also one's interface with the broader social world—a place to welcome guests or a retreat when the world feels threatening or over-whelming. The environment of one's home is so foundational that it only stands to reason that housing and mental health would be linked. But how do we best understand these links empirically? In the literature to date, two themes have emerged to describe the human experience of housing: tenure and stability on the one hand and housing quality on the other. Tenure refers to the possession or occupation of housing, and stability implies predictable, long-term tenure of housing in some form or another. Quality, on the other hand, refers to the housing itself: its materials, environmental control systems (ventilation, heating, cooling), and other physical attributes. We also might consider the quality of the neighborhood more broadly, including socioeconomic issues such as poverty or residential segregation, as well as physical features such as the aggregate upkeep of building infrastructure and the presence of public facilities and services. Interpreted broadly in this way, housing stability and quality address much of what is important about housing's role in mental health, not to mention much of the scope of federal housing policy.

With housing being a fundamental human need, it is not surprising that those who experience homelessness—at the extreme end of the spectrum of housing instability—face myriad health problems. Individuals experiencing homelessness have higher rates of mental illnesses, substance use, trauma, injury, suicide, and virtually every other marker of poor mental health and well-being (Fazel et al. 2008). This relationship is bidirectional: those with mental health and substance use issues are at higher risk for economic marginalization, unemployment, isolation, and, ultimately, homelessness; however, there is also strong evidence that homelessness itself is toxic to mental health (Fazel et al. 2014).

The *loss* of housing is a serious trauma that has impacts on mental health, whether or not it results in chronic homelessness. Eviction, for example, is an increasingly widespread phenomenon, particularly among Black families (Desmond 2012). Research has shown that eviction may place mothers at sustained risk for depression (Desmond and Kimbro 2015). Similarly, foreclosure, the loss of ownership of a home due to inability to pay one's mortgage, is associated with deterioration in mental and physical health (Tsai 2015).

Although homelessness is the most striking and visible extreme on the spectrum of housing tenure, individuals who face other, less visible forms of housing instability (e.g., doubling up, falling behind on rent, couch surfing) are at risk as well (Taylor 2018). Unaffordable housing has the potential to affect people in several ways, regardless of whether they end up unhoused, by constraining resources for other expenditures, inducing chronic stress, and increasing the risk of reduced socioeconomic status (Lorant 2003). The problem of cost burden—paying more than 30% of one's gross income on housing expenses—is extremely widespread, affecting just under half of renters and a quarter of homeowners in 2019 (Joint Center for Housing Studies of Harvard University 2019).

Although relatively few studies have examined the relationship between housing burden and health, there is evidence to support the idea that excessive housing cost burden may be detrimental to mental health (Baker et al. 2020). If unstable or unaffordable housing can precipitate mental distress, it stands to reason that housing support could improve mental health and well-being, a proposition supported by evidence showing improved mental health outcomes and reduced health expenditures for people placed into permanent housing, particularly when those programs offer the support necessary to meet their often complex needs (Hunter et al. 2017). What about the larger federal programs we spent much of this chapter examining? HUD's Family Options Study demonstrated that housing-unstable families who were able to procure long-term housing subsidies through the Section 8 program reported improved health and well-being over time, as well as greater housing stability (Gubits et al. 2018).

Unfortunately, because federal housing and rent subsidies are in short supply, large numbers of eligible families remain on long waiting lists. The data we have reviewed make plain the cost at which we underresource these programs, but what is the cost of the psychological effect of enduring such prolonged waiting periods despite knowing that one is eligible for support? The answer is not empirically understood; however, given that waiting is the default position of so many families in need of support, the experience and its impacts certainly deserve further study.

Apart from affordability and stability, housing quality has long been a concern of federal housing policy as well, although not always for the good: urban renewal stemmed in large part from concerns over the perceived quality of housing and neighborhoods. Although urban renewal is no longer official federal policy, governments, public health researchers, urbanists, and community members alike are as much as ever concerned with the quality—physical and social—of urban neighborhoods. Validating this interest, a good deal of recent work substantiates the idea that mental health is influenced by the home and neighborhood environments.

Some elements of the physical housing environment, including proper ventilation and surrounding green space, are linked to improved well-being and mental health (Ige et al. 2019). Lower-quality housing and lack of green space, by contrast, are associated with depression (Rautio et al. 2018), and particular noxious elements have been linked to poor mental health outcomes, including psychological distress from overcrowding and noise, negative affect from malodorous air pollutants, and often serious cognitive and behavioral problems from key toxins such as lead (Evans 2003; Rollings et al. 2017). Interventional research has supported the value of physical upgrades to housing. For example, efforts to improve building quality have yielded mental health benefits, including improvements in quality of life from heating and energy efficiency upgrades (Thomson et al. 2009) and a greater ability to use housing for social purposes (which are mental health promoting) following housing renovation (Fullilove et al. 1999). The physical quality of the neighborhood as a whole has also been implicated in outcomes such as depression (Mair et al. 2008), although empirical results related to regeneration efforts at the neighborhood level have been more mixed, perhaps because of the potential for subsequent exclusion following improvements through processes such as gentrification (Tulier et al. 2019).

What about the neighborhood as a social environment? In recent years, this has become a subject of great interest to researchers, although the idea that the degree of social cohesion in a community is relevant to mental health is not a new one. For example, more than a half century ago the researchers of the Stirling County Study observed that socially cohesive communities had lower rates of psychiatric problems compared with less cohesive communities (Leighton et al. 1963). One commonly studied construct for conceptualizing social cohesion is *collective efficacy*. This term refers to both the strength of social cohesion in a community (*collective*) and its members' ability to achieve goals and shape community norms and behavior (*efficacy*) (Sampson 2012). Collective efficacy is a property of communities, one whose positive psychological effects are well supported by research. For example, collective efficacy is linked to lower rates of substance use (Vaeth et al. 2015), lower rates of anxiety and depression in adolescents (Donnelly et al. 2016), reduced rates of PTSD following a natural disaster (Fullerton et al. 2019), and lower rates of violent crime (Sampson 1997). Moreover, it seems that collective efficacy may mediate some of the observed relationship between socioeconomic disadvantage and poor mental health (Xue et al. 2005). Unfortunately, federal policy has often done considerable harm to collective efficacy in urban communities, particularly communities of color. A variety of policies, including redlining, racially discriminatory home mortgage insurance policies, urban renewal, HOPE VI, and mass incarceration, have contributed to urban racial segregation and, subsequently, to the repeated destabilization, dismantling, and displacement of Black neighborhoods (Fullilove and Wallace 2011; Rothstein 2017). In particular, mass incarceration not only disrupts communities but can prohibit future access to public housing for justice-involved individuals. These policies' negative impact on the stability and cohesion of Black neighborhoods over time is dramatic (Fullilove 2005; Izenberg and Fullilove 2016).

The role of the federal government has not been universally detrimental, however. Federal housing assistance has demonstrated the potential to provide stability and thus offer recipients the chance to form social connections and develop social support in their communities (Clampet-Lundquist 2010). Numerous federal policies, the 1965 Housing Act among them, have helped to fund community organizations and facilities, greenspace, transit, the arts, and other community-building and community-sustaining programs. Since 1968, housing discrimination has been against the law, although in practice federal enforcement has often been lacking and exclusion persists in legal forms, such as through zoning codes that ostensibly have nothing to do with race but, in fact, have the effect of disproportionately preventing people of color from moving to certain neighborhoods (Rothstein 2017).

Future of U.S. Housing

From deadly protests in Watts to the committed leadership of Robert Weaver, U.S. housing policy—which is also mental health policy—has been characterized by both turbulence and an often unclear path forward. Strides have been made, but the journey is not complete. As of this writing, the United States remains in a housing crisis. Cost burden is extraordinarily widespread, particularly among economically vulnerable people. Indeed, as of 2016, roughly half of all U.S. renters were cost burdened, defined as spending more than 30% of their gross income on rent (Hobbes 2018). This crisis ultimately comes down to a gap between supply and demand: the United States' more than 11.4 million extremely low income households have access to only 7.5 million affordable rental units, about half of which (3.5 million) are already rented to higher-income households (Boghani 2017). A complicated web of factors has led to this situation, including massive cuts to investment in public and affordable housing programs during the 1980s, the loss (through demolition, renovation, and upgrade) of more than 2.5 million affordable units since 1990 (Hobbes 2018), a financial crisis that cut wages and pushed millions of homeowners back into the rental market (Covert 2018), and the lasting economic effects of the coronavirus SARS-CoV-2 disease (COVID-19) pandemic. All of this has occurred in the context of rising income inequality, a shrinking social safety net, and ongoing resistance to affordable housing construction in many communities.

Despite the vast need, hostility to federal housing efforts has remained a viable strategy in American politics. Ben Carson, secretary of HUD under President Donald J. Trump, suggested early on in his tenure that dependence on public benefits such as housing assistance was a major problem (Gonzalez 2016) and went so far as to advocate for funding cuts at his own department (Boburg 2017) while reducing the amount of federal housing aid given to qualifying families (Board 2018). The faltering commitment to housing under the Trump administration was not just about federal funding; during this time HUD also largely abandoned a mission that had historically been at its core: the investigation of and enforcement against discriminatory housing practices (Thrush 2018).

Although threats to HUD diminished under the administration of President Joseph R. Biden, it is worth hypothesizing for a moment about their potential impact because they could become reality again before long. Cuts to HUD would likely reduce the already small proportion of qualifying families able to obtain housing assistance and squeeze the incomes of those lucky enough to get a subsidy to begin with, ultimately increasing the risk of cost burden and allowing housing costs to cut even deeper into other essential expenditures such as health care and food. This would no doubt increase the rate of evictions and homelessness. Although a growing number of states and local municipalities are enacting nondiscrimination laws (Bell et al. 2018), a scaling back of federal fair-housing enforcement would undermine efforts to mitigate decades of residential segregation and could heighten the already substantial barriers to residential integration facing those who receive housing assistance.

Starting in the latter half of the 2010s, a number of legislators began to respond to the housing crisis with proposals seeking to directly address the issue. As examples, then Senator Kamala Harris of California offered the Rent Relief Act, and Senator Cory Booker of New Jersey proposed the Housing, Opportunity, Mobility, and Equity Act. Both bills continued the trend of focusing on rent subsidies rather than the construction of new housing. However, unlike previous bills, both offered refundable tax credits going straight to renters, thereby addressing what has become a major limitation of the Section 8 Housing Choice Voucher Program and a source of ongoing discrimination, namely, finding a landlord willing to accept a voucher (Sullivan and Anderson 2017). At least one analysis suggested that these bills could produce massive reductions in poverty (Matthews 2019).

Taking a somewhat different approach, Senator Elizabeth Warren of Massachusetts introduced a bill known as the American Housing and Economic Mobility Act of 2018. This far-reaching proposal offered to put $45 billion dollars a year for 10 years into the housing trust fund, a relatively new program designed to subsidize the construction and preservation of affordable housing (Anzilotti 2018). But beyond simply encouraging housing construction, Senator Warren's bill sought to address decades of racial housing segregation by attacking the local zoning laws that perpetuate housing discrimination: under the bill, a series of community development grants would be made available to municipalities under the condition that their zoning laws comply with best practices in nondiscrimination. Finally, the act offered down payment assistance targeted to groups, such as people of color, who have historically been excluded from home ownership. Senator Warren's legislation was arguably most like the housing omnibus bills of the mid-twentieth century, insofar as it sought to tackle housing insecurity from multiple angles at once. Some estimates suggested the bill could lower rents nationwide by 10% over 10 years (Anzilotti 2018).

Renovating the House of Federal Policy

Federal housing policy is like a historic home adapting to meet the needs of each new family residing there. A home is built just once, but to continue to serve its residents in the long term, it must be maintained, repaired, renovated, revised, and, often, expanded over time. The Housing Act of 1965 was not the foundation or the original frame. It *was* a major renovation that, along with subsequent renovations, has left us with a house that scarcely resembles the original. Today's version is in some ways better but in other ways as flawed as ever and sorely in need of investment. At the time of this writing, it is hard to say exactly what the next revision of federal housing policy will look like, although the proposals described above offer some promising ideas. It is a near certainty, however, that no matter when these words are being read, housing policy will need yet another update.

The important link between housing and mental health must be one lens through which we interrogate the next revision to federal housing policy, whenever we may find it on the legislative agenda. We can imagine the questions we might ask: Does this law reduce the burden of housing costs and thus the risk of eviction and foreclosure? Does it support those on the path out of housing instability and homelessness, or does it place demands on them? Is it large enough to help all those who need it, or will it yet again subject many to interminable wait lists? Does it realize higher-quality and more affordable options for people at every income level, or does it favor those with higher incomes? Does it reduce residential segregation and exclusion or reinforce them? Does it foster strong, connected, and vibrant neighborhoods, or does it encourage their fracturing through displacement or gentrification? Does it ultimately help lift families out of poverty? If it seeks to be good medicine, future housing policy must provide satisfactory answers to these questions.

References

Anzilotti E: Elizabeth Warren has a plan to help end the housing crisis. Fast Company, 2018. Available at: www.fastcompany.com/90242320/elizabeth-warren-has-a-plan-to-help-end-the-housing-crisis. Accessed February 16, 2022.

Baker E, Lester L, Mason K, et al: Mental health and prolonged exposure to unaffordable housing: a longitudinal analysis. Soc Psychiatry Psychiatr Epidemiol 55(6):715–721, 2020 32140739

Bell A, Sard B, Koepnick B: Prohibiting discrimination against renters using housing vouchers improves results. Washington, DC, Center on Budget and Policy Priorities, December 20, 2018. Available at: www.cbpp.org/research/housing/prohibiting-discrimination-against-renters-using-housing-vouchers-improves-results. Accessed February 16, 2022.

Biles R: Public housing and the postwar urban renaissance, 1949–1973, in From Tenements to the Taylor Homes: In Search of an Urban Housing Policy in Twentieth Century America. Edited by Bauman JF, Biles R, Szylvian KM. University Park, Pennsylvania State University Press, 2000, pp 143–163

Board LTE: What homeless crisis? HUD Secretary Ben Carson wants to raise rents on the poorest of the poor. Los Angeles Times, April 27, 2018. Available at: www.latimes.com/opinion/la-ed-hud-housing-20180427-story.html. Accessed February 16, 2022.

Boburg S: Trump seeks sharp cuts to housing aid, except for program that brings him millions. The Washington Post, June 20, 2017. Available at: www.washingtonpost.com/investigations/trump-seeks-sharp-cuts-to-housing-aid-except-for-program-that-brings-him-millions/2017/06/20/bf1fb2b8-5531-11e7-ba90-f5875b7d1876_story.html. Accessed February 16, 2022.

Boghani P: A housing affordability crisis that's worse for the lowest income Americans. PBS Frontline, May 9, 2017. Available at: www.pbs.org/wgbh/frontline/article/a-housing-affordability-crisis-thats-worse-for-the-lowest-income-americans. Accessed February 16, 2022.

Brauer CM: Kennedy, Johnson, and the War on Poverty. J Am Hist 69(1):98, 1982

Center on Budget and Policy Priorities: Policy basics: the housing choice voucher program. Washington, DC, Center on Budget and Policy Priorities, 2017a. Available at: www.cbpp.org/sites/default/files/atoms/files/PolicyBasics-housing-1-25-13vouch.pdf. Accessed February 16, 2022.

Center on Budget and Policy Priorities: Policy basics: project based rental assistance. Washington, DC, Center on Budget and Policy Priorities, 2017b. Available at: www.cbpp.org/research/housing/section-8-project-based-rental-assistance. Accessed February 16, 2022.

Center on Budget and Policy Priorities: Policy basics: public housing. Washington, DC, Center on Budget and Policy Priorities, 2021. Available at: www.cbpp.org/sites/default/files/atoms/files/policybasics-housing.pdf. Accessed February 16, 2022.

Clampet-Lundquist S: "Everyone had your back": social ties, perceived safety, and public housing relocation. City Community 9(1):87–108, 2010

Covert B: The deep, uniquely American roots of our affordable housing crisis. The Nation, 2018. Available at: www.thenation.com/article/give-us-shelter/. Accessed February 16, 2022.

Curtis MA, Garlington S, Schottenfeld LS: Alcohol, drug, and criminal history restrictions in public housing. Cityscape: A Journal of Policy Development and Research 15(3):37–52, 2013

Desmond M: Eviction and the reproduction of urban poverty. A J Sociol 118(1):88–133, 2012

Desmond M, Kimbro RT: Eviction's fallout: housing, hardship, and health. Social Forces 94(1):295–324, 2015

Donnelly L, McLanahan S, Brooks-Gunn J, et al: Cohesive neighborhoods where social expectations are shared may have positive impact on adolescent mental health. Health Aff (Millwood) 35(11):2083–2091, 2016 27834250

Evans GW: The built environment and mental health. J Urban Health 80(4):536–555, 2003 14709704

Fazel S, Khosla V, Doll H, et al: The prevalence of mental disorders among the homeless in western countries: systematic review and meta-regression analysis. PLoS Med 5(12):e225, 2008 19053169

Fazel S, Geddes JR, Kushel M: The health of homeless people in high-income countries: descriptive epidemiology, health consequences, and clinical and policy recommendations. Lancet 384(9953):1529–1540, 2014 25390578

Folkart BA: Marquette Frye, whose arrest ignited the Watts riots in 1965, dies at age 42. Los Angeles Times, December 25, 1986. Available at: www.latimes.com/archives/la-xpm-1986-12-25-me-486-story.html. Accessed February 16, 2022.

Fullerton CS, Mash HBH, Wang L, et al: Posttraumatic stress disorder and mental distress following the 2004 and 2005 Florida hurricanes. Disaster Med Public Health Prep 13(1):44–52, 2019 30616708

Fullilove MT: Root Shock: How Tearing Up City Neighborhoods Hurts America and What We Can Do About It. New York, Random House, 2005

Fullilove MT, Wallace R: Serial forced displacement in American cities, 1916–2010. J Urban Health? 8 (3) 81 –389, 2011 21607786

Fullilove MT, Green L, Fullilove RE: Building momentum: an ethnographic study of inner-city redevelopment. Am J Public Health 89(6):840–844, 1999 10358672

Gershon L: Did the 1965 Watts riots change anything? JSTOR Daily, July 13, 2016. Available at: https://daily.jstor.org/did-the-1965-watts-riots-change-anything. Accessed February 16, 2022.

Gonzalez S: Future HUD secretary Ben Carson '73 stresses self-sufficiency as goal of government programs. Yale News, December 9, 2016. Available at: https://news.yale.edu/2016/12/09/future-hud-secretary-ben-carson-73-stresses-self-sufficiency-goal-government-programs. Accessed February 16, 2022.

Gubits D, Shinn M, Wood M, et al: What interventions work best for families who experience homelessness? Impact estimates from the Family Options Study. J Policy Anal Manage 37(4):735–766, 2018 30272428

Hobbes M: America's housing crisis is a ticking time bomb. Huffington Post, 2018. Available at: www.huffingtonpost.com/entry/housing-crisis-inequality-harvard-report_us_5b27c1f1e4b056b2263c621e. Accessed February 16, 2022.

Housing and Urban Development Act of 1965, Pub. L. 89-117, 79 Stat. 451.

Hunter S, Harvey M, Briscombe B, et al: Evaluation of Housing for Health permanent supportive housing program. Santa Monica, CA, RAND Corporation, 2017. Available at: www.rand.org/pubs/research_reports/RR1694.html. Accessed February 17, 2022.

Ige J, Pilkington P, Orme J, et al: The relationship between buildings and health: a systematic review. J Public Health (Oxf) 41(2):e121–e132, 2019 30137569

Izenberg JM, Fullilove MT: Hospitality invites sociability, which builds cohesion: a model for the role of main streets in population mental health. J Urban Health 93(2):292–311, 2016 26955815

Jacobs J: The Death and Life of Great American Cities. New York, Vintage Books, 1961

Joint Center for Housing Studies of Harvard University: The state of the nation's housing. Cambridge, MA, Joint Center for Housing Studies of Harvard University, 2019. Available at: www.jchs.harvard.edu/sites/default/files/Harvard_JCHS_State_of_the_Nations_Housing_2019.pdf. Accessed February 16, 2022.

Kerner Commission: Report on the National Advisory Commission on Civil Disorders. Washington, DC, U.S. Government Printing Office, 1968

Krock A: In the nation: paying other people's rent. The New York Times, May 27, 1965. Available at: https://timesmachine.nytimes.com/timesmachine/1965/05/27/97203521.html?pageNumber=36. Accessed February 16, 2022.

Leighton DC, Harding JS, Macklin DB, et al: Psychiatric findings of the Stirling County study. Am J Psychiatry 119:1021–1026, 1963 13929431

Leopold J, Getsinger L, Blumenthal P, et al: The housing affordability gap for extremely low-income renters in 2013. Washington, DC, The Urban Institute, June 15, 2015. Available at: www.urban.org/sites/default/files/publication/54106/2000260-The-Housing-Affordability-Gap-for-Extremely-Low-Income-Renters-2013.pdf. Accessed February 16, 2022.

Lorant V: Socioeconomic inequalities in depression: a meta-analysis. Am J Epidemiol 157(2):98–112, 2003 12522017

Mair C, Roux AVD, Galea S: Are neighbourhood characteristics associated with depressive symptoms? A review of evidence. J Epidemiol Community Health 62(11):940–946, 2008 18775943

Martin Luther King, Jr. Research and Education Institute: Watts Rebellion (Los Angeles). Stanford, CA, The Martin Luther King, Jr., Research and Education Institute, Stanford University, June 5, 2018. Available at: https://kinginstitute.stanford.edu/encyclopedia/watts-rebellion-los-angeles. Accessed February 16, 2022.

Matthews D: Cory Booker and Kamala Harris's affordable housing plans, explained. Vox, February 2, 2019. Available at: www.vox.com/future-perfect/2019/2/2/18205913/rent-kamala-harris-cory-booker-poverty. Accessed February 16, 2022.

Mazzara A: Housing vouchers work: huge demand, insufficient funding for housing vouchers means long waits. Washington, DC, Center on Budget and Policy Priorities, April 19, 2017. Available at: www.cbpp.org/blog/housing-vouchers-work-huge-demand-insufficient-funding-for-housing-vouchers-means-long-waits. Accessed February 16, 2022.

National Low Income Housing Coalition: The long wait for a home. Housing Spotlight, 2016. Available at: https://nlihc.org/sites/default/files/Housing Spotlight_6-1_int.pdf. Accessed February 16, 2022.

Parson D: The decline of public housing and the politics of the red scare. Journal of Urban History 33(3):400–417, 2016

Pritchett WE: Robert Clifton Weaver and the American City. Chicago, IL, University of Chicago Press, 2008

Rautio N, Filatova S, Lehtiniemi H, et al: Living environment and its relationship to depressive mood: a systematic review. Int J Soc Psychiatry 64(1):92–103, 2018 29212385

Rollings KA, Wells NM, Evans GW, et al: Housing and neighborhood physical quality: children's mental health and motivation. J Environ Psychol 50:17–23, 2017

Rothstein R: The Color of Law. New York, Liveright, 2017

Sampson RJ: Neighborhoods and violent crime: a multilevel study of collective efficacy science. Science 277(5328):918–924, 1997 9252316

Sampson RJ: Great American City: Chicago and the Enduring Neighborhood Effect. Chicago, IL, University of Chicago Press, 2012

Scally CP, Batko S, Popkin SJ, et al: The case for more, not less: shortfalls in federal housing assistance and gaps in evidence for proposed policy changes. Washington, DC, The Urban Institute, January 2018. Available at: www.urban.org/sites/default/files/publication/95616/case_for_more_not_less_1.pdf. Accessed February 16, 2022.

Schwartz AF: Housing Policy in the United States, 3rd Edition. New York, Routledge, 2014

Semple R: $7.5 billion bill, with rent subsidy proviso, signed by Johnson. The New York Times, August 11, 1965. Available at: www.nytimes.com/1965/08/11/archives/75-billion-bill-with-a-rent-subsidy-proviso-signed-by-johnson-75.html. Accessed February 16, 2022.

Sugrue TJ: The Origins of the Urban Crisis: Race and Inequality in Post War Detroit. Princeton, NJ, Princeton University Press, 1996

Sullivan L, Anderson M: Section 8 vouchers help the poor—but only if housing is available. NPR, May 10, 2017. Available at: www.npr.org/2017/05/10/527660512/section-8-vouchers-help-the-poor-but-only if-housing-is-available. Accessed February 16, 2022.

Taylor LA: Housing and health: an overview of the literature. Health Affairs, June 7, 2018. Available at: www.healthaffairs.org/do/10.1377/hpb20180313.396577/full/. Accessed February 16, 2022.

Thomson H, Thomas S, Sellstrom E, et al: The health impacts of housing improvement: a systematic review of intervention studies from 1887 to 2007. Am J Public Health 99(suppl 3):S681–S692, 2009 19890174

Thrush G: As affordable housing crisis grows, HUD sits on the sidelines. The New York Times, July 27, 2018. Available at: www.nytimes.com/2018/07/27/us/politics/hud-affordable-housing-crisis.html. Accessed February 16, 2022.

Tsai AC: Home foreclosure, health, and mental health: a systematic review of individual, aggregate, and contextual associations. PLoS One 10(4):e0123182, 2015 25849962

Tulier ME, Reid C, Mujahid MS, et al: "Clear action requires clear thinking": a systematic review of gentrification and health research in the United States. Health Place 59:102173, 2019 31357049

Vaeth PAC, Caetano R, Mills BA: Binge drinking and perceived neighborhood characteristics among Mexican Americans residing on the U.S.-Mexico border. Alcohol Clin Exp Res 39(9):1727–1733, 2015 26247487

von Hoffman A: High ambitions: the past and future of American low-income housing policy. Hous Policy Debate 7(3):423–446, 1996

von Hoffman A: Let us continue: housing policy in the Great Society, part one. Cambridge, MA, Joint Center for Housing Studies of Harvard University. April 1, 2009. Available at: www.jchs.harvard.edu/research-areas/working-papers/let-us-continue-housing-policy-great-society-part-one. Accessed February 16, 2022.

von Hoffman AA: A study in contradictions: the origins and legacy of the Housing Act of 1949. Housing Policy Debate 11(2):299–326, 2010

Weaver RC: Human values of urban life. Proc Acad Polit Sci 27(1):31–39, 1960

Xue Y, Leventhal T, Brooks-Gunn J, et al: Neighborhood residence and mental health problems of 5- to 11-year-olds. Arch Gen Psychiatry 62(5):554–563, 2005 15867109

9 | Learning From History's Lessons

How Mental Health Professionals Can Participate in Policy Change

Michael T. Compton, M.D., M.P.H.
Marc W. Manseau, M.D., M.P.H.

By highlighting seven federal laws, we have shown that non-health-related legislation affects social determinants of health and social determinants of mental health. Given that nearly every policy influences one or more social determinant, all policies are health policies, and all policies are mental health policies. Whether it is policy related to early childhood programs, education, civil liberties, employment, income, taxation, energy, housing, food, farming, transportation, infrastructure, the environment, immigration, or war and other forms of conflict, it is fair to assume that there are built-in, although usually unrecognized or

The authors are grateful for the review and very helpful input provided by Julie Suarez at Cornell University's College of Agriculture and Life Sciences.

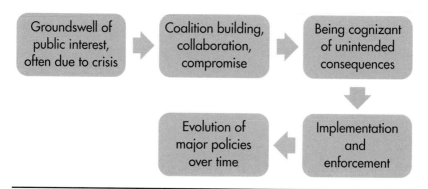

FIGURE 9–1. **Five facets of policy change.**

minimally considered, health impacts. Those health impacts can be substantial, sustained, and, importantly, inequitably distributed unless measures are in place to ensure equity and justice. As we have seen through seven examples—although countless others could be described—at the population level, policy widely and substantially affects health, including mental health, both positively and negatively. Mental health promotion and mental illness prevention occur through policy change; here, we have seen that such policy change can relate to farming economic policy, labor and union organizing policy, income security policy, environmental conservation policy, civil rights and antidiscrimination policy, education quality policy, and housing policy. Now, we conclude with some final observations and thoughts about how policy change occurs and how mental health professionals can be involved in this process.

Lessons Learned About Past (Passed) Federal Legislation and Mental Health

We can identify a number of recurring themes across the seven chapters covering our seven prototypical major federal laws that shaped social determinants of mental health and thus influenced mental health in America. Here, we distill them to five facets of policy change (Figure 9–1).

Public Interest

Many major legislative acts are initially conceived through a groundswell of public interest, often in response to a crisis. Although the seven acts reviewed in this volume moved forward and were ultimately enacted through the legislative (political, policymaking) process, their need and intent were initially conceived because of problems that were being increasingly recognized in society. The National Labor Relations Act of 1935, for example, came about not just because of congressional interest in the issue but because of investigative journalism and a growing awareness of the problem of child labor, gross exploitation of workers, and major inequalities in income and wealth. The increasing interest led to mass public actions and, ultimately, to breaking points, such as massive strikes against poor working conditions, employers using overtly violent methods to scare employees into returning to work, and the 1894 Pullman railroad strike and boycott that brought travel to a halt in most of the Midwest. As another example of a groundswell of public interest, decades later, growing discontent about racism and Jim Crow policies resulted in nonviolent civil disobedience, including sit-ins at the Woolworth's lunch counter in Greensboro, North Carolina, and the Freedom Rides on buses departing the nation's capital and heading southward. Peaceful protests were all too often violently confronted by local law enforcement. Congress and the president had to act. Protests spurred action and resulted in the eventual passage of the Civil Rights Act of 1964.

Coalition Building

All major legislative acts are birthed from coalition, collaboration, and compromise. Opposing sides must come together for the greater good, be willing to see others' viewpoints, and be willing to compromise and put some desired policy change elements on hold. Coalition building is the method for accumulating sufficient support and, ultimately, enough votes. Often, discussions about the process of making legislation are too simplified into which political parties have more power. Even when one political party holds a majority, unless it has a very numerically steep majority such as during the New Deal flurry of legislative activity in the 1930s, the process of enacting policy requires coalition building among colleagues both within and outside the same political party.

Coalition building is often a difficult and painstaking process, and it usually involves years (sometimes lifetimes) of work organizing various interest groups and stakeholders. But it is a key ingredient of policymaking. In terms of mental health impacts of policies, part of coalition building is about having the right allies (which can include psychiatrists and other mental health professionals) and having the right information (which psychiatrists and other mental health professionals can help to provide).

We have seen coalition building, collaboration, and compromise in the seven featured federal acts. As Rexford Tugwell, part of Roosevelt's Brains Trust, was helping to craft the Agricultural Adjustment Act of 1933, not all experts believed that the Title I voluntary domestic allotment approach would work, yet enough conceded and agreed to try it in light of the desperate circumstances. We saw in the story of the Clean Air Act of 1963 that Edmund Muskie canvassed numerous environmental activist groups and masterfully balanced their interests with those of key industry leaders and then collected and included the best suggestions of his colleagues. As such, the Clean Air Act reflected Senator Howard Baker's belief that technology could be harnessed to reduce air pollution, Senator Tom Eagleton's commitment to deadlines as a necessary ingredient of laws that would deliver on promises, and Muskie's own insistence that environmental law safeguard human health. Like Muskie, accomplished policymakers know when to walk away from negotiations to force concessions and how to collaborate effectively.

As mental health professionals are well aware, coalition, collaboration, and compromise are really about relationships. One's ability to make change is largely dependent on the strength of one's own relationships, which includes integrity, credibility, trustworthiness, and empathy. Although political scientists carry out extensive research trying to quantify the impact of money on politics or the affects of grassroots movements and petitions on politics and policy, the reality is that relationships tend to matter the most. They can be long-term, personal ones, or they can be transactional and fleeting, but in the end, policy is decided by individual human beings and groups of human beings in relationships with one another. In seeking to use our influence in the policymaking realm, we must be prepared with the understanding that change takes a long time and is best accomplished through a network of relationships built over time—either within advocacy groups or trade associations that employ professional lobbyists or from working with elected officials and regulatory officials directly. Despite today's tendency toward social media, actual, direct human interactions remain the best way to effectuate public policy change; it helps when the information provided is clear, factual, and based on science.

Unintended Consequences

We also saw that nearly all policies, even those generally promoting mental health, have unintended—initially unrecognized or ignored—consequences that can be less mental health promoting or can even worsen mental health for some groups. American history is replete with structural racism influencing policy. For example, with regard to the Agricultural Adjustment Act of 1933, the first Farm Bill, sharecroppers and tenant farmers, who were more likely to be African American, were clearly disadvantaged; the first Social Security Act also excluded much of this same population from disability benefits. Although this inequity was partly addressed in subsequent iterations, attention to equity in the nutrition title of the Farm Bill has entered into the policymaking process only in recent decades, and discussions about racial equity in the distribution of agricultural or farmer subsidies in the Farm Bill have come into public consciousness only over the past decade. Similarly, provisions in the National Labor Relations Act of 1935 failed to adequately protect workers of color, beginning a legacy of racial discrimination in American labor organizing that has only recently abated. Now unions do more to boost wages for people of color than other groups, and union membership is associated with reduced racism in white workers. The Housing and Urban Development Act of 1965 did not correct—and instead perpetuated—the racially motivated activity of urban renewal, in which localities would use federal money to seize swaths of "blighted" neighborhoods, raze them, displace the people who lived there, and redevelop the land for other uses. Thousands of such projects across the nation targeted for destruction many thousands of homes and neighborhoods—overwhelmingly those of people of color—rather than providing investment for actual renewal.

Some of these unintended consequences might actually be "intended" because of the entrenched history of structural racism in American society. Racism is a "system of oppression that is based in and upholds the superiority of white people and the inferiority of Black, Indigenous, and People of Color. Racism is created by and upheld through policies, practices, and procedures to create inequities between racial groups" (National League of Cities 2020). As such, *antiracism* is also a system: "a system in which we create policies, practices, and procedures to promote racial equity" (National League of Cities 2020). Policies, including federal acts, must be intentionally structured around antiracism, or else they will likely continue to be structured by racism.

Implementation and Enforcement

Passage of the law is just the first step; implementation and responsible governance are what really count. Laws without implementation and enforcement are nothing more than words on a piece of paper. Each of the laws that we reviewed in this volume would have had no teeth without appropriations. The passage of a law does not mean the goal is accomplished; in fact, many laws on the books are simply ignored because funding did not follow. Among the laws highlighted here, in some cases, entire federal departments or agencies would have to be established, which meant new employees and new policies, processes, and regulations. Budgets would need to be developed and monitored. New programs would require oversight and ongoing assessment. Consider the Social Security Act of 1935. Although the law itself is a remarkable work product, the real work in changing America and improving health and mental health resides within the array of benefits programs operated by the Social Security Administration, an independent federal agency with roughly 60,000 employees at its headquarters in Maryland, 10 regional offices, 8 processing centers, and more than 1,000 field offices across the country.

Decades later, the Clean Air Act of 1963 was monumental, but its implementation and governance were and continue to be what really matter: national research and development programs, regional air pollution programs, new technology and energy sources, and enforceable standards for the automotive industry and other diverse types of American companies. Much of this implementation and enforcement ends up being political in nature, molded by the ever-shifting governing philosophies and ideological perspectives of presidential administrations and subject to pressures and influences from various interest groups, including corporate lobbyists and advocacy organizations. Therefore, in order to confer sustained benefits to health and mental health, organizing and advocacy efforts must not end with the enactment of a particular law but rather must continue indefinitely.

The courts also play a role in implementation of policies. Environmental policy, for example, has been strongly influenced by district courts and the Supreme Court, which up until recently have upheld the ability of the Environmental Protection Agency (EPA) to have broad rule-making authority and discretion in establishing regulatory dictates over issues ranging from pesticide registration to methane emissions from oil and gas. However, the recent Supreme Court ruling in *West Virginia v. EPA* (West Virginia v. EPA 597 U.S. 1126 [2022]) calls into serious question the extent to which the EPA will continue to be able to regulate greenhouse gas emissions, likely necessitating further Congressional action to combat the existential threat of climate change.

Evolution of Policies

We have observed and demonstrated that all major policies evolve over time. Improvements are made, amendments are added, and titles are restructured. This may occur as a gradual evolution over time or in fits and starts depending on how coalitions are able to make progress (e.g., which parties hold the White House, House of Representatives, and Senate). For example, 30 years after the Elementary and Secondary Education Act of 1965 set a standard for eliminating "separate but equal" educational practices, its iterations over time have moved the nation closer to the ideal goal of all students having access to high-quality public education. As another example of policy evolution, after the Social Security Act of 1935 created a foundation, many of its programs expanded in the ensuing decades to cover more people and to provide more generous benefits. Sometimes laws are made less helpful or even harmful to health and mental health, such as further revisions to the Social Security Act that restructured public assistance programs under "welfare reform" in the 1990s.

Role for Psychiatrists and Other Mental Health Professionals

It could be said that mental health professionals' roles have become very circumscribed (largely because of the need to deliver treatment efficiently and how the work of our professions is financed) to individual-level patient care (e.g., prescriptions, psychotherapy), which might have powerful effects for individuals but does little to nothing to improve the mental health of entire populations. Nonetheless, mental health professionals can have a role in each of the five aspects of policymaking. That is, we can instigate or contribute to the groundswell of public interest often needed to ignite policy change, including lawmaking; be involved in organizing efforts, including coalition building; help to ensure that unintended consequences such as those driven by structural racism are eliminated; see that implementation occurs in such a way that mental health is, indeed, promoted; and observe and contribute to a law's evolution over time. We can do all of these things through writing and presenting, working with the professional organizations and health care institutions with which we are affiliated (which often represent respected and even powerful interest groups), participating in a public hearing or forum, giving testimony, connecting directly with elected officials at the state or federal level, and contributing our perspective and expertise to the work of advocacy groups that are doing critical organizing work on the ground. Although our focus here has been on federal policy (in particular, very large federal acts that substantially shaped both American life and, as we argue, the mental health of the population), policymaking obviously also occurs at the state level.

Getting involved even more locally—at the local city or county level, or within even smaller jurisdictions (such as towns, townships, villages, hamlets)—can also be rewarding and have impact. However, for the most part, local governmental jurisdictions simply implement social service policies in which the state or federal government gives them an active role. For example, many counties help administer social services locally, but the state controls the policymaking process. At the town and village level, local decision-making is largely confined to such issues as maintaining roads; dealing with permits for animals, residential building projects, and the like; and handling business planning issues such as whether or not local leaders can attract a business to the town. As such, relative to federal and state policymaking, far less policy is actually done at the local level that is significant in terms of affecting population mental health.

In terms of the observation that many policies are initially conceived through a groundswell of public interest, often in response to a crisis, mental health professionals can help to shift social norms so that mental health implications are recognized. We can voice our opinions, both as professionals with content expertise and also as citizens with our own personal stake in the outcome of diverse types of policies. We can use our voices to bolster the voices of those who might otherwise be suppressed, such as the patients we serve and their families—while fully respecting patient privacy laws and all ethical standards—with special attention to those affected by long-standing structural racism and other forms of social injustice.

With regard to the initial birthing of a policy via coalition, collaboration, and compromise, mental health professionals can be at the table as part of the coalition or collaborative. Because mental health is so uncommonly a consideration in the policy deliberation process, we cannot necessarily expect to be invited. We have to ask to be there. Thankfully, chances are that as physicians, psychologists, other licensed mental health professionals, and certified paraprofessionals, we will be welcomed and our input will be valued. Furthermore, as experts in interpersonal relationships, group dynamics, and conflict and compromise, we might have a role in facilitating successful coalition building. So here in this facet of policymaking, mental health professionals might bring both content expertise and process expertise.

Along those same lines, the third facet of policymaking that we consistently observed across our case studies of federal acts was that unintended consequences—initially unrecognized or ignored—can be less mental health promoting or can even worsen mental health for some groups. Here, too, psychiatrists and other mental health professionals can be part of scouring policies—at the institutional, organizational, local, state, and federal levels—for inequities. This should be a valued function of the mental health professions because the existence of inequities undoubtedly sets the stage for adverse social determinants of mental health, which in turn negatively affect the mental health of the population.

Just as mental health professionals can be involved in the passage of a law, so too can they be at the table during its implementation and oversight. Through professional organizations and advocacy groups or on their own, mental health professionals can contribute to the initial rule making of executive agencies by submitting official comments. With the advent of the internet, along with open meetings laws intended to promote sunshine in government and transparency, much of the policymaking process that was once obscure to average citizens with day jobs is now easily accessible. The federal government and most state governments have relatively accessible online platforms that frequently have recorded public hearings and show calendars of legislation being considered along with pertinent committee meetings. Regulatory agencies publish their draft rules and have opportunities to comment on their websites. A simple internet search will often yield a treasure trove of information about how to participate in various policymaking settings.Mental health professionals can also provide expertise in considering the mental health implications of the implementation process, ensuring maximal mental health benefits. As a law takes effect over time, mental health professionals can help monitor whether the law is having the intended effects and can speak out when they notice lackluster mental health benefits or even mental health harms. In addition, we can watch carefully for proposed changes to regulations and enforcement when new presidents, governors, and federal and state legislators take office, and we can advocate for or against proposed changes to implementation.

We also note that all major policies evolve over time. Our participation in a law's evolution might be the most important step we can take. Once a bill passes and a law is securely in place, what can policymakers do to tweak it to improve its positive mental health impacts over time or reduce its unintended harms? Many citizens believe that once a law passes it is irrefutable. The reality is that laws and policy evolve, not just with interpretations by the courts and through regulatory processes but also by simple amendment of the law over time. It is even possible (although highly difficult) to amend the U.S. Constitution, as the slow but steady (and as yet unsuccessful) process of moving toward adoption of the Equal Rights Amendment exemplifies. Mental health professionals should avoid becoming discouraged and should recognize that we all can have a voice and a role.

Collaborating With Policymakers and Advocacy Groups and Conducting Mental Health Impact Assessments

Policymakers often need content expertise beyond that of their staff. Here, we are referring to expertise in potential unforeseen mental health impacts of laws and policies that have nothing, at face value, to do with mental health. Such expertise can take the form of a formal evaluation—a mental health impact assessment, as described below—but is often needed more urgently on an ad hoc basis. Unlike the yearslong time frame of traditional research or even an in-depth impact assessment, policymakers often need to make decisions that cannot be delayed until research is produced and published (Khatana et al. 2017).

Although letting your voice be heard can occur over the phone, by email or letter, or via social media, physicians also have opportunities for more direct engagement. Meeting with a member of Congress (or their staff) or a member of the state legislative body (or their staff) is a highly effective way to discuss specific issues or legislative priorities, and guidance on how to go about doing that is available (American Medical Association 2022).

Collaborating on policy change requires a game plan. In contrast to clinical practice, academic research, teaching, health care management and leadership, and various combinations of those activities, no clear career pathway exists for psychiatrists and other mental health professionals to engage in public policymaking. Additionally, policy work is usually not a reimbursable service, and the opportunity costs of reduced clinical, research, or teaching output are a barrier for physicians considering public policy involvement (Khatana et al. 2017). Given these obstacles, it can be easy for mental health professionals to lose sight of our social responsibility to promote mental health and prevent mental illnesses. This dilemma likely occurs in other social service sectors as well; for example, food bank staff and managers have become so concerned with the mechanics of getting food to food insecure people that they have arguably lost sight of their social responsibility to advocate for an end to the need for food banks (Fisher 2017). Mental health professionals should be advocating for policies that will have preventive effects in addition to their ongoing work in the clinical or treatment setting.

Pathways to prepare for and engage in policy work have been outlined and include such approaches as joint degree programs (e.g., in public health or public policy); involvement with local and national physicians' organizations; electives, away rotations, and fellowships during training; and executive and leadership training programs (Khatana et al. 2017). Mental health professionals can also seek mentoring and supervision from established advocates and lobbyists, just as we seek mentoring and supervision for our clinical work.

Beyond individual connections to policymakers, psychiatrists and other mental health professionals can join the forces of advocacy groups, either within the health care field or outside it. Advocacy groups specifically for health care professionals exist for nearly all policy areas, spanning, for example, from general health care advocacy (e.g., Doctors for America, Physicians for a National Health Program) to human rights and social justice (e.g., Physicians for Human Rights, Physicians for Social Justice) to gun violence prevention (e.g., Doctors 4 Gun Safety, Psychiatrists for Gun Violence Prevention) to global climate change (e.g., The Medical Society Consortium on Climate and Health, Climate Psychiatry Alliance). Countless other advocacy groups exist for the general public (i.e., membership is not structured by profession or vocation) on every issue imaginable, and many, if not most, would welcome the perspective and expertise of mental health professionals. When mental health professionals do decide to join advocacy organizations, it is important to balance sharing expertise with humbly allowing other members—who may have personal life experience with the issue or decades of dedication to the cause—to lead the efforts and campaigns. In our academic or clinical careers, pressure and necessity to exhibit leadership often exist given our roles and training, as well as the need for measurable achievement to advance our careers. When collaborating with activists and other advocates, it is often preferable to listen and contribute in ways in which we are asked to, rather than attempting to take over and control the strategies and activities. In essence, finding community and solidarity with like-minded advocates should often be prioritized over seeking public recognition or taking credit for initiatives. Over time, as we gain experience and detailed knowledge about the issue at hand and the communities affected, we can allow for leadership opportunities to emerge naturally.

For upcoming policy decisions that will have an extended time frame, a more formal, in-depth analysis of the positive and negative mental health implications can be informative and productive. *Health impact assessments* are systematic evaluations that use a variety of data sources and analytic methods to assess the potential health impacts of proposed policies, plans, programs, and projects in various sectors (Dannenberg 2016). Although the number of health impact assessments has increased in recent decades, few systematically consider mental health impacts, and very few have specifically addressed mental health. The process has been formalized (as the Mental Wellbeing Impact Assessment [MWIA]) by the South London and Maudsley National Health Service Foundation Trust and partners in the United Kingdom as a stepwise process that begins with a desk-based screening tool and culminates in a workshop that engages multiple stakeholders and results in coproduced action plans (Cooke et al. 2011). Todman and colleagues (2012) have also formalized the process in the United States.

As an example of a *mental health impact assessment*, Todman et al. (2012) analyzed the effect of a proposed amendment to Chicago's Vacant Buildings Ordinance on the collective mental health of people living in Englewood, a neighborhood located on the city's southwest side. At the time, 712 foreclosed properties were listed in Englewood. Major elements of the proposed amendment were to expand the definition of a property *owner* to include banks and other entities that initiate foreclosure proceedings on vacant properties, to impose higher fees and fines on owners of five or more properties who maintain vacant properties, to require that owners of five or more properties post a $10,000 bond for each vacant property, and to pay a 5% finder's fee to city residents who reported building code violations. Goals of the amendment were to ensure that the city is paid quickly for the fees and fines it assesses, to create incentives for residents to help identify violations of the Vacant Buildings Ordinance, and to ensure that more properties are secured and maintained. The impact assessment determined that a number of social determinants would be affected, including those pertaining to safety and reduced crime and violence, enhanced employment opportunities, local economic activity, public services, collective efficacy, civic engagement, and trust (Todman et al. 2012). Beneficial impacts on depression, anxiety, and substance use were identified that likely would not have otherwise been considered.

Todman and coworkers (2013) also evaluated the mental health impact of proposed changes to the U.S. Equal Employment Opportunity Commission Policy Guidance, again in Englewood, Chicago. Specifically, they asked, "What is the impact on the mental health of a community when employers use arrest records in making employment decisions about members of that community?" Through a highly iterative process involving literature reviews and dialogues with Englewood residents, they identified four social determinants most likely to be affected by the Equal Employment Opportunity Commission revision to disallow use of arrest records: social exclusion (i.e., the systematic marginalization of groups of people within a society), employment, income, and neighborhood conditions, each of which has important links to individual- and community-level mental health. They predicted a potential moderate to substantial increase in the employability of Englewood residents, as well as possibly other communities with large numbers of residents with arrest records. Given the distributional effects of this and the accompanying beneficial mental health impacts, the policy change was evaluated as resulting in some measure of restorative equity; that is, it would reduce mental health inequities.

Pope and colleagues (L.G. Pope, D.J. Pohl, A. Ehntholt, et al.: "New York State's Bail Elimination Act of 2019: A Mental Health Impact Assessment," submitted for publication) conducted a retrospective mental health impact assessment of New York State's Bail Elimination Act of 2019, which eliminated money bail and mandated pretrial release for most misdemeanors and nonviolent felonies, which make up approximately 90% of all arrests statewide. They assessed the likely impact of the law on individuals who would otherwise be detained on a pretrial basis with regard to nine social determinants, ranging from adverse childhood experiences to access to health care. Although the law had already been enacted, the impact assessment may inform other states' policymaking in the area of criminal justice reform and could also affect the ongoing implementation of and evolution of this policy in New York. As noted earlier, the passage of a law does not mean that it is irrefutable; most laws evolve over time. Mental health professionals can help shed light on what aspects of the law help versus harm a community's mental health. Despite some progress in the area of mental health impact assessment, as exemplified by these three diverse examples, much more work needs to be done in formalizing and initiating the process for analyzing policies spanning diverse sectors of society.

Shaping Mental Health in America

As we have seen, psychiatrists and other mental health professionals have, in addition to their vital roles in serving patients in clinical settings and advancing the science and practice of treatment for mental illnesses, an opportunity to contribute to policy that affects social determinants of mental health and thus affects the mental health of the population. Whatever one's social justice–related interest, whether it be racism, educational inequality, poor housing, food insecurity, urban design problems, or the worsening condition of the environment, there is a role to engage in ongoing policymaking. Furthermore, policymakers are often unlikely to consider the mental health impacts of non-health policies—those impacts must be clearly pointed out by mental health professionals or public health professionals with a keen interest in mental health.

This work also shifts the focus from one of tertiary prevention (treatment aimed at reducing disability) to one of primary prevention. As such, the mental health professions have an opportunity to engage in activities that will reduce the risk of (and thus prevent) mental illnesses and substance use disorders altogether, in addition to promoting the mental health of all members of the population by helping to create a more equal, just, and peaceful society that meets everyone's basic needs and fosters less trauma. It will require struggle at times and solidarity at other times, but the end goal of promoting mental health will be worth the effort.

References

American Medical Association: Congressional check-up: a guide to physician advocacy. Chicago, IL, American Medical Association, 2022. Available at: www.ama-assn.org/sites/ama-assn.org/files/corp/media-browser/public/washington/communicating-with-congress_0.pdf. Accessed February 18, 2022.

Cooke A, Friedli L, Coggins T, et al: MWIA: A Toolkit for Well-Being, 3rd Edition. London, National MWIA Collaborative, 2011

Dannenberg AL: Effectiveness of health impact assessments: a synthesis of data from five impact evaluation reports. Prev Chronic Dis 13:E84, 2016 27362932

Fisher A: Big Hunger: The Unholy Alliance Between Corporate America and Anti-Hunger Groups. Cambridge, MA, MIT Press, 2017

Khatana SAM, Patton EW, Sanghavi DM: Public policy and physician involvement: removing barriers, enhancing impact. Am J Med 130(1):8–10, 2017 27555096

National League of Cities: What does it mean to be an anti-racist? Washington, DC, National League of Cities, July 21, 2020. Available at: www.nlc.org/article/2020/07/21/what-does-it-mean-to-be-an-anti-racist. Accessed May, 28, 2021.

Todman L, Hricisak LM, Fay JE, et al: Mental health impact assessment: population mental health in Englewood, Chicago, Illinois, USA. Impact Assessment and Project Appraisal 30(2):116–123, 2012

Todman L, Taylor JS, McDowell T, et al: U.S. Equal Employment Opportunity Commission policy guidance: a mental health impact assessment. Chicago, IL, Institute on Social Exclusion, Adler School of Professional Psychology, April 2013. Available at: www.pewtrusts.org/~/media/Assets/2013/04/01/ArrestRecordsinEmploymentDecisions.pdf. Accessed October 25, 2021.

Index

Page numbers printed in **boldface** type refer to tables or figures.